YOGA
AT HOME

LIZ LARK AND MARK ANSARI

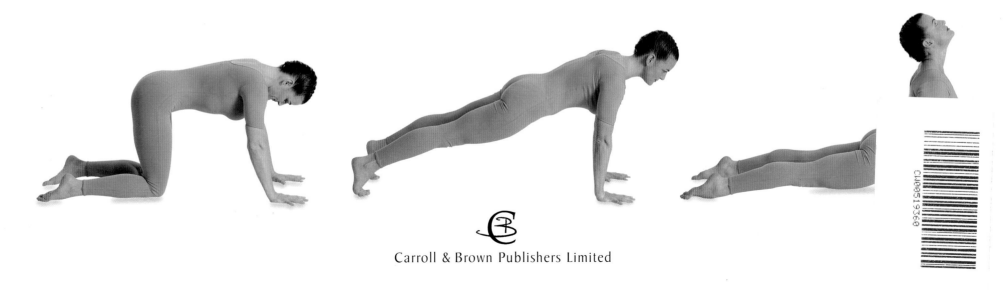

Carroll & Brown Publishers Limited

This edition published in 2008 in the United Kingdom by

Carroll & Brown Publishers Limited
20 Lonsdale Road
London NW6 6RD

Text © Liz Lark and Mark Ansari 1998, 2008
Illustrations and compilation © Carroll & Brown Limited 1998, 2008

Previously published in 1999 in the United Kingdom as *Yoga for Beginners* by Newleaf

A CIP catalogue record for this book is available from the British Library.

ISBN 978-1-904760-69-6

10 9 8 7 6 5 4 3 2 1

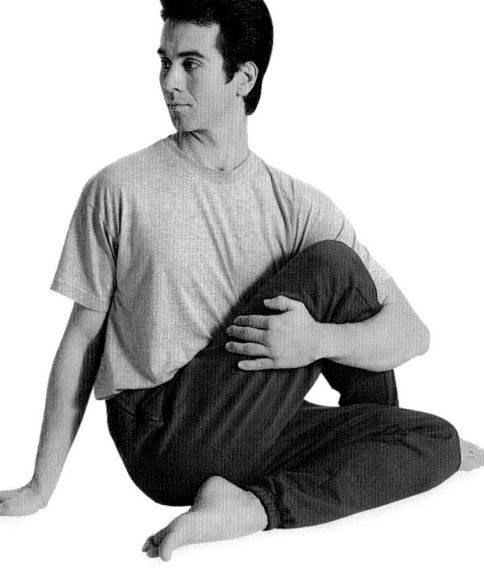

Printed and bound in China by Leo Paper Products Ltd

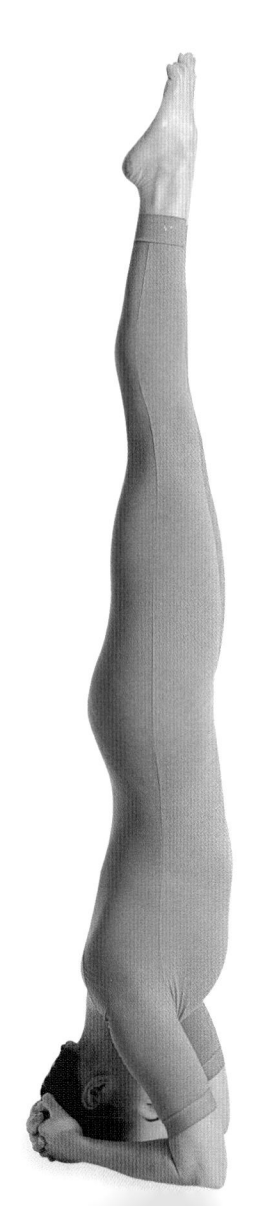

FOREWORD

Yoga teaches us to relax physically, focus our minds and keep our problems in perspective. It also helps to counteract the stresses and strains of the modern world, making it the perfect antidote to the rapidly changing pace of our busy lives.

Yoga helps you achieve harmony between your body and mind. The practice of poses (known as *asanas*) and breathing exercises (*pranayama*) cleanses your body, restores your energy and makes you stronger and more flexible; it will also enable you to achieve emotional balance, leaving you better equipped to deal with the demands of your lifestyle.

Yoga at Home is a practical guide intended to introduce you safely and accessibly to the basic postures, breathing techniques and other practices of yoga. You don't need any previous experience of yoga: the easy-to-follow instructions make this guide suitable for the complete novice or anyone wishing to supplement their yoga practice at home. The book includes two series of exercises. Once you are thoroughly familiar with the postures and techniques of the beginner's programme you can move on to the slightly more advanced intermediate programme.

We have found that yoga has enhanced our lives remarkably, not only by changing our bodies, but also by opening the doors to an exciting journey of self-discovery. We hope that our book will enable you, too, to feel the benefits of stretching, moving and breathing freely for yourself as you relieve built-up stress, learn to relax and ultimately get more out of your day-to-day life. Enjoy!

LIZ LARK AND MARK ANSARI

CONTENTS

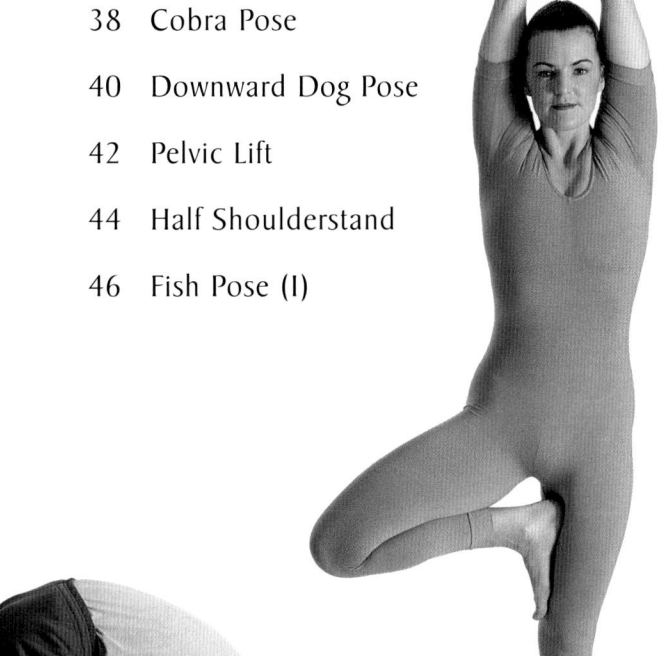

Intermediate Program

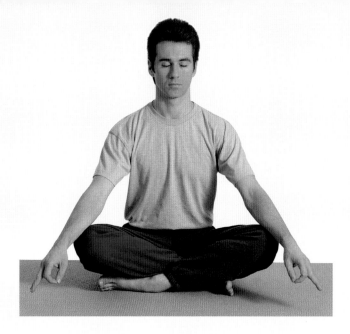

The Yoga Way of Life

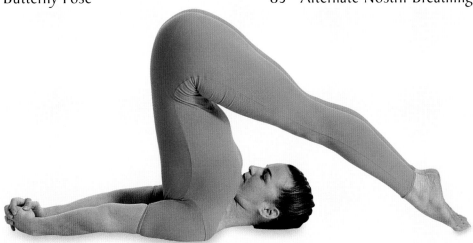

PREPARING FOR PRACTICE

The word yoga comes from the Sanskrit root yuj, *meaning yoke or union. The aim of this ancient Eastern practice is to create unity between the self and the outer world, and to resolve inner turmoil in order to help us achieve our full potential.*

Regular yoga practice creates harmony between the mind and the body. This calms the disorder of our thoughts—as if stilling the ripples on a lake—so that we better perceive our connection to the world around us.

HATHA YOGA There are many forms of yoga, the most well known being *hatha yoga*, which literally translates from Sanskrit as "union through determined effort." Hatha yoga uses the discipline of physical postures and breathing techniques to "yoke" the body to the mind, thus opening a pathway to physical health, emotional stability, and mental balance.

The benefits of this ancient yoga practice are recorded in many writings, including the sacred Hindu texts of the *Upanishads* and the *Bhagavad Gita,* which date from between 400 and 200 BC. The contemporary practice of hatha yoga is based largely on a medieval text called the *Yoga Sutras of Patanjali* (see page 86).

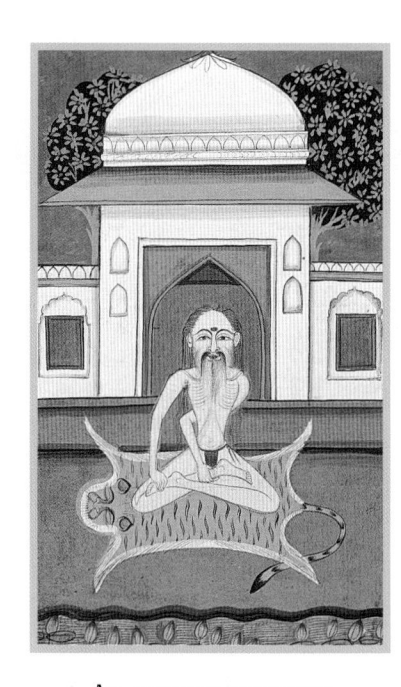

AN ANCIENT DISCIPLINE
Yoga has been practiced throughout India for millennia. This eighteenth-century Punjabi painting depicts a yogi performing his daily *asanas.*

TAPPING OUR TRUE POTENTIAL The basic principle of yoga is that the key to happiness resides within each of us. The practice of yoga is simply the means by which we discover and draw upon this innate wisdom. Yoga opens the door to our full potential as individuals through a system of conscious exercise that trains not only the body but also the breath and, ultimately, the mind.

Yoga for Beginners is an introductory guide to some of the basic postures (*asanas*) and breathing techniques (*pranayama*) of this fascinating system of conscious exercise. It includes two complete, well-balanced yoga routines—a beginner's and an intermediate program—which can be followed for daily practice.

But yoga is more than just a series of exercises, and at the end of the book you will find an introduction to some of the philosophical principles that make yoga a whole way of life.

BEFORE YOU BEGIN With proper care and preparation, yoga is a safe, effective, and rewarding activity that is suitable for people of all ages and from all walks of life. But to make your yoga practice as fulfilling and enjoyable as possible, it's best to observe the following simple guidelines.

Try as far as possible to perform your postures at the same time each day. Not only will this ensure steady progress, but it is also a good way to develop a sustainable daily routine that will help you achieve long-lasting and positive results.

Choose a time that is convenient for you, when you won't be distracted by other commitments. Early morning, late afternoon, or early evening are all suitable times. Some people find they are quite stiff first thing in the morning, but your energy levels are at their highest at this time of the day. A warm shower before you begin will help loosen your muscles and joints.

At the end of the day, you may have less energy and find it harder to concentrate, but your muscles and joints will be looser and this will make your practice easier. Early evening is also a good time for a yoga session and will help you to unwind. It will also improve the quality of your sleep.

Whatever time of the day you choose, always be sure to practice yoga on an empty stomach. Allow an interval of at least two hours to digest any meal you have eaten, and ideally, empty your bowels and bladder before you begin your *asanas*.

THE RIGHT ENVIRONMENT Whether you perform your postures inside or outdoors, make sure your practice area is quiet, comfortable, and warm. It should have a flat (but not too hard) surface with sufficient room for you to stretch in all directions and a good supply of fresh air. The ideal yoga environment is somewhere you won't be disturbed, and preferably a place that you find conducive to a serene, elevating frame of mind.

When practicing, try to expose as much skin to the air as possible and make sure that your clothing does not restrict your movement. Most yoga teachers advise that you perform your *asanas* in bare feet. Remove your watch, glasses, and any jewelry before you begin.

Try not to leave your designated practice area or otherwise interrupt your session. If you need props such as a block or pillows, make sure they are within easy reach before you begin. To cushion your back, knees, and other parts of your body, use a yoga mat, a large towel, or a neatly folded blanket.

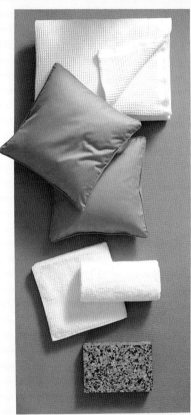

BASIC REQUIREMENTS
A mat or blanket and possibly cushions or a yoga block are all you will need to practice yoga.

Relaxation

When we experience stress, our nervous system allows us to cope by stimulating the body to work at a more intense level. But long periods of stress can cause a damaging build-up of tension. The tonic for all of this is relaxation: it promotes physical, mental, and emotional health.

THE EFFECTS OF RELAXATION When you are relaxed, your parasympathetic nervous system counters the effects of stress by slowing your breathing and heart rate. Your emotional condition is also eased as you move from your normal waking state (the beta state) to a level that is even deeper and more beneficial than sleep (the alpha state). Yoga helps you achieve this alpha state, slowing down your brain activity and restoring your physical and mental vitality, thereby enabling you to recover from the pace of your daily life.

An ideal time to relax is directly before and after your yoga workout. The classic relaxation posture is called *Savasana*, the Corpse Pose. In this supine position, your breathing deepens and your heart rate slows, increasing the flow of oxygen to every part of your body and releasing built-up tension from your joints and muscles.

8

THE CORPSE POSE
The sensation of profound stillness is what gives the Corpse Pose its name. You may feel very drowsy in this posture but try to remain awake so you are conscious of the beneficial physical and mental sensations.

--- TAKE CARE ---

Come out of Savasana very slowly and gently. Roll onto your side and rest before getting up.

▼ *If you suffer from backache, raise your legs onto a chair or lie in a semi-supine position.*

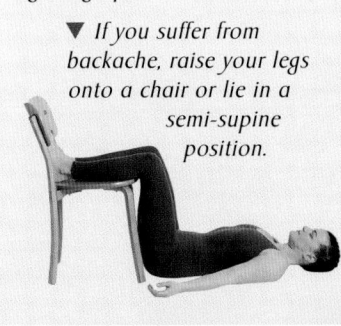

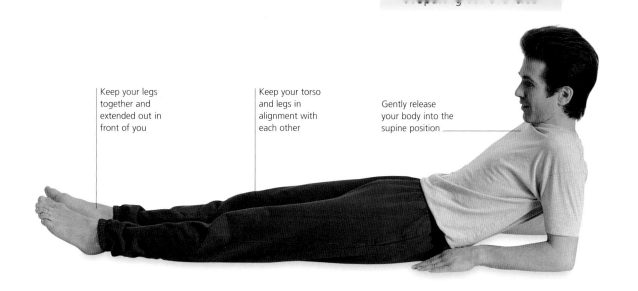

Keep your legs together and extended out in front of you

Keep your torso and legs in alignment with each other

Gently release your body into the supine position

1 Sit on the floor, stretch your legs out in front of you with your feet together, and lean back onto your elbows. Come down gently into a fully supine position, release any tension in your back, and stretch out through your arms, legs, spine, and neck.

2 Extend your neck and press your chin toward your chest. Draw your shoulders away from your ears, press your lower back into the floor by angling your tailbone upward, push your buttocks away from your sacrum (the five fused vertebrae at the base of your spine), and press into the floor with your hands.

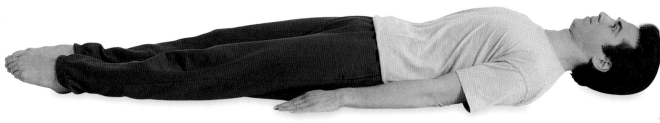

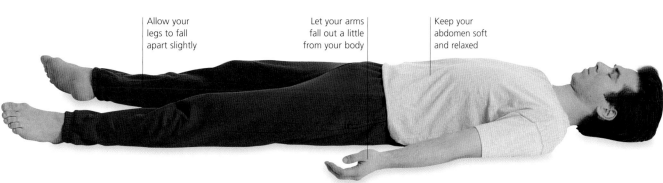

Allow your legs to fall apart slightly

Let your arms fall out a little from your body

Keep your abdomen soft and relaxed

3 Turn the palms of your hands up and extend your arms. Relax your face and feel your body sinking into the floor. Close your eyes and mentally scan your body, adjusting any areas that are out of alignment on either side of your spine. Turn your attention inward, breathe quietly and easily, and try to be as still as possible.

* *Hold posture for 5 minutes.*

The Complete Yoga Breath

Your state of mind is reflected in the way you breathe. If you are nervous or stressed, your breathing will be rapid and shallow. But when you relax, you sigh, let go, and breathe deeply. Most adults do not breathe to their full capacity and the insufficient supply of oxygen to the body contributes to their fatigue and stress.

THE BENEFITS OF BREATHING The classic breathing exercise shown here is called the Complete Yoga Breath. It develops good habits by increasing your awareness of the sensations of your breath in the three key locations of your torso: shallow in the clavicular top chest, stronger in the thorax, and deepest in the abdomen.

The Complete Yoga Breath forms an integral part of the relaxation at the end of each workout, but it is also essential to breathe properly *throughout* your practice, so you may find it useful to begin your practice with this breathing exercise as well. This not only increases the intake of oxygen as you inhale and eliminates toxins such as carbon dioxide as you exhale, but also massages and tones the internal organs as your diaphragm moves up and down with each breath. Focusing on your breathing calms your thoughts and makes the mind steady, while the increased amount of oxygen reaching your brain improves your concentration.

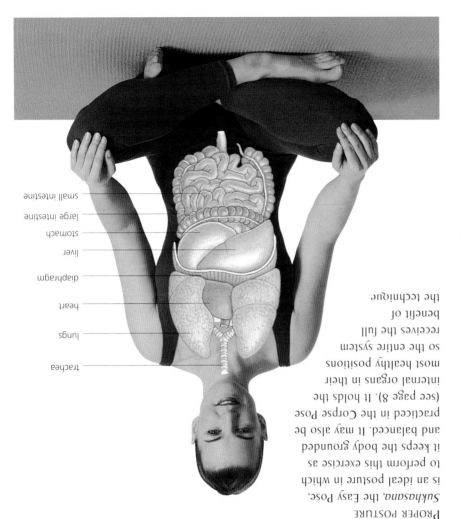

trachea

lungs

heart

diaphragm

liver

stomach

large intestine

small intestine

PROPER POSTURE
Sukhasana, the Easy Pose, is an ideal posture in which to perform this exercise as it keeps the body grounded and balanced. It may also be practiced in the Corpse Pose (see page 8). It holds the internal organs in their most healthy positions so the entire system receives the full benefit of the technique.

10

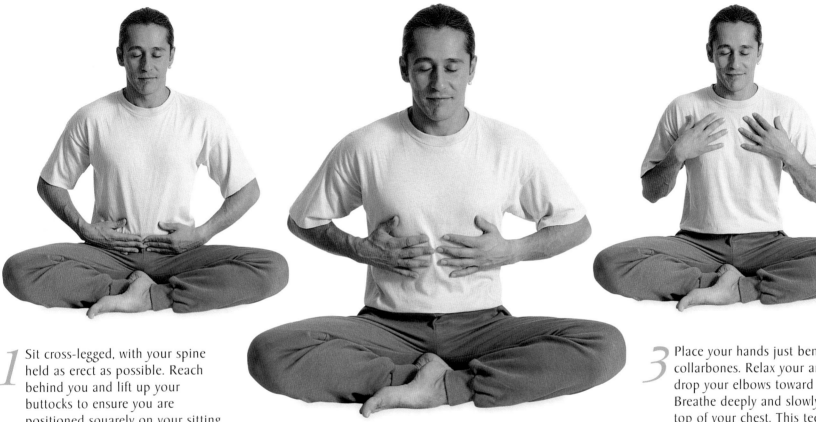

1 Sit cross-legged, with your spine held as erect as possible. Reach behind you and lift up your buttocks to ensure you are positioned squarely on your sitting bones. Extend up through your spine to lengthen the back of your neck and lift your head. Open your chest and relax your shoulders. Place your hands on your abdomen, below the navel. Breathe deeply so that your hands rise and fall slowly in time with your breath.

▷ *Continue for 10 breaths.*

2 Place your hands on your ribcage and breathe slowly and deeply. As you inhale, your ribcage expands and your diaphragm moves down to massage your abdominal organs. As you exhale, your ribcage deflates and your diaphragm moves up to give your heart a gentle massage.

▷ *Continue for 10 breaths.*

3 Place your hands just beneath your collarbones. Relax your arms and drop your elbows toward the floor. Breathe deeply and slowly into the top of your chest. This technique increases awareness of the breath, expands and deepens the thorax, and encourages your lungs to take in oxygen to their full capacity.

▷ *Continue for 10 breaths.*

Limbering Up

To prepare yourself for the practice of your *asanas*, it's vital that you perform a set of limbering postures beforehand, especially if you are new to yoga. These will increase mobility of the skeletal system, invigorate the muscles and internal organs, and encourage mental relaxation. Limbering up warms the body systems by increasing the circulation of blood to the muscles. It also releases tension in the spine and loosens any stiffness in the major joints.

The following preparatory stretches heighten physical responsiveness and gently improve flexibility before the more rigorous demands of your workout. The posture shown below is particularly helpful for relieving trapped wind and expelling impurities from the digestive system. Try always to spend 10–15 minutes limbering up before your yoga practice. This also helps to reduce the possibility of injury caused by inadequate preparation.

WIND RELIEVING POSE

Beginning in the Corpse Pose, inhale, stretch your arms over your head, and point your toes. Bring your right leg up, bend your knee, and clasp your shin with both hands. Gently squeeze your right thigh into your abdomen, keeping your neck and shoulders relaxed. This opens the hip joint and sacrum and also works the muscles of the thigh.

✳ *Hold for 10 breaths.*

▷ *Repeat 5 times with alternate legs.*

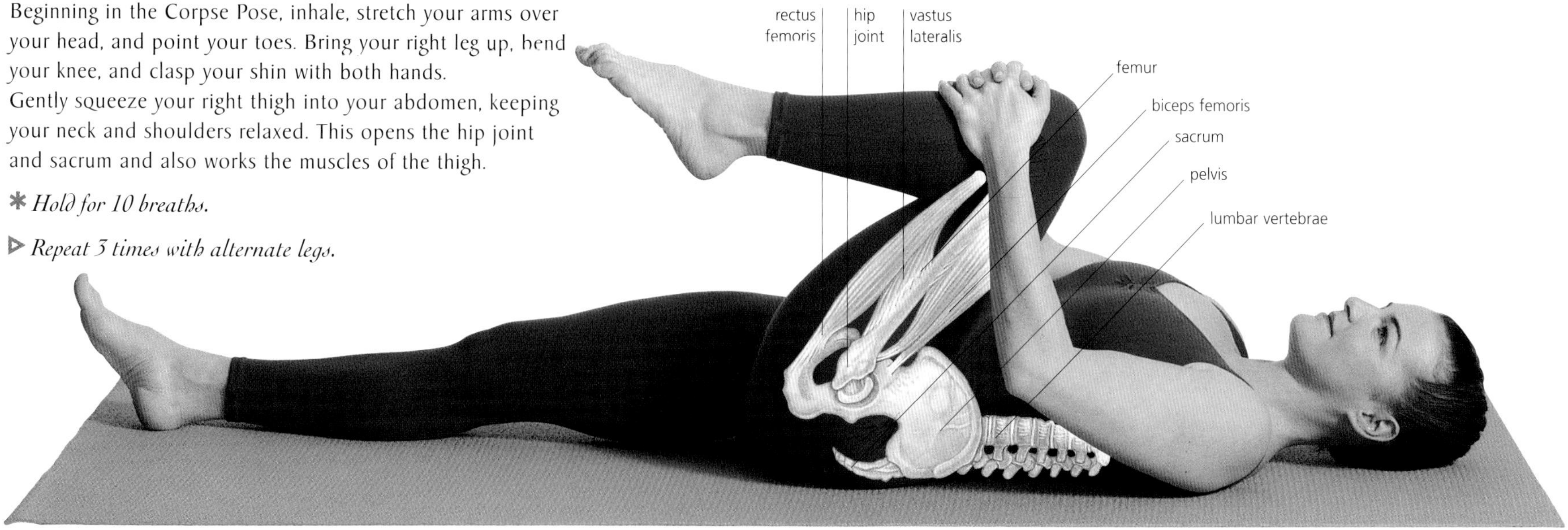

lumbar vertebrae

pelvis

sacrum

biceps femoris

femur

vastus lateralis

hip joint

rectus femoris

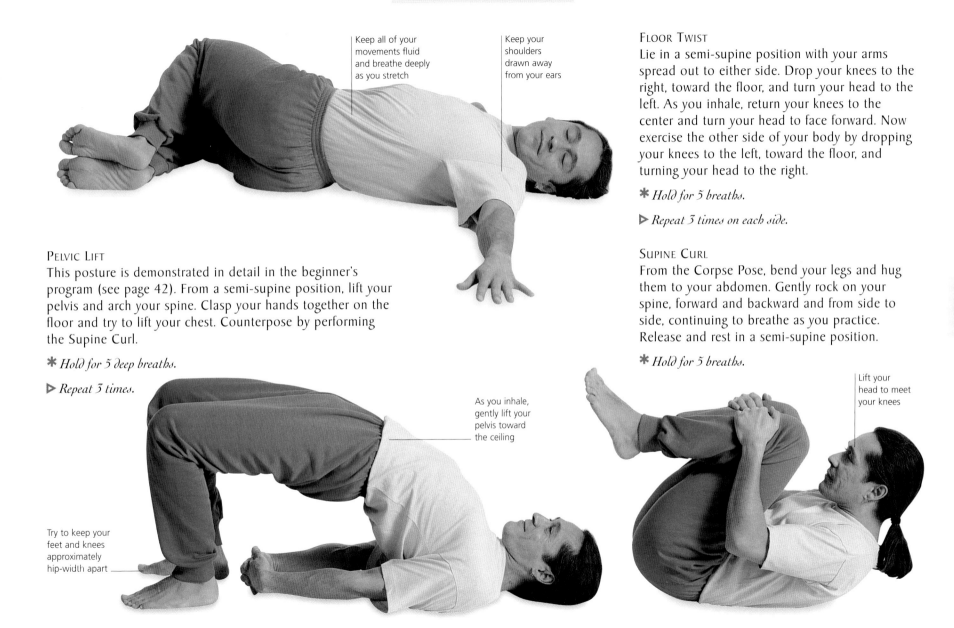

Keep all of your movements fluid and breathe deeply as you stretch

Keep your shoulders drawn away from your ears

Floor Twist

Lie in a semi-supine position with your arms spread out to either side. Drop your knees to the right, toward the floor, and turn your head to the left. As you inhale, return your knees to the center and turn your head to face forward. Now exercise the other side of your body by dropping your knees to the left, toward the floor, and turning your head to the right.

✱ *Hold for 5 breaths.*

▷ *Repeat 3 times on each side.*

Pelvic Lift

This posture is demonstrated in detail in the beginner's program (see page 42). From a semi-supine position, lift your pelvis and arch your spine. Clasp your hands together on the floor and try to lift your chest. Counterpose by performing the Supine Curl.

✱ *Hold for 5 deep breaths.*

▷ *Repeat 3 times.*

Supine Curl

From the Corpse Pose, bend your legs and hug them to your abdomen. Gently rock on your spine, forward and backward and from side to side, continuing to breathe as you practice. Release and rest in a semi-supine position.

✱ *Hold for 5 breaths.*

13

As you inhale, gently lift your pelvis toward the ceiling

Lift your head to meet your knees

Try to keep your feet and knees approximately hip-width apart

Awakening the Spine

Your general health is reflected by your posture and the condition of your spine. Much of the tension of daily life is stored in this area, and consequently manifests itself in stiff back muscles and aching neck and shoulders. A sedentary lifestyle, slumped stance, and a general lack of activity all contribute to back problems.

GENTLE PREPARATION Yoga can help you achieve a strong and flexible spine. However, without proper limbering, a tense and unresponsive back can make it impossible to practice certain postures comfortably and correctly. It's important, therefore, to gently awaken the spine during your warm-up. If you are taking a yoga class, inform the teacher of any condition affecting your back so that he or she can advise you of the best postures to perform.

The Cat Pose is a gentle way to exercise your spine. In this posture your back should be gently curved. Focus on synchronizing the upward arch and subsequent dip of the spine with deep breaths. This will help you to achieve the fluid, cat-like movements that give this posture its name.

THE CAT POSE
This dynamic limbering sequence of movements places a healing stretch through the entire length of the back and encourages the circulation of healthy blood from the base of the spine to the head. It also has a calming influence on the mind.

1 Lie in *Darnikasana*, the Child Pose, and relax your shoulders, neck, and face. Breathe deeply and slowly into your lower abdomen and feel it press against your thighs. This posture helps to develop abdominal breathing.

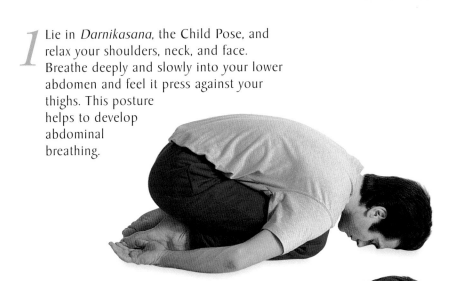

2 Lift your hips toward the ceiling and roll onto the crown of your head, into the Raised Child Pose. Keep your arms relaxed and feel the gentle stretch in the back of your neck. Focus on the expansion in the upper part of your ribcage as you fill your lungs on an inhalation. This posture develops thoracic breathing.

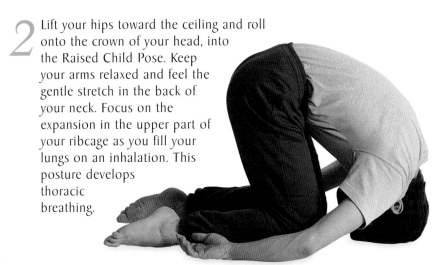

15

3 Come onto all fours with your hands directly beneath your shoulders and your knees aligned with your hips. Inhale, look up, dip your spine, and stretch your tailbone toward the ceiling. Breathe into the top of your chest to help develop clavicular breathing.

✳ *Hold for 10 breaths.*

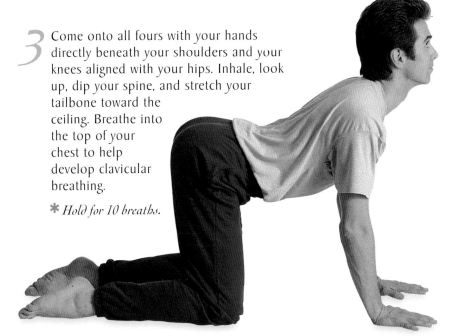

4 Continuing to breathe into the top of your ribcage, exhale, squeeze your chin to your chest, arch your spine, and tuck in your tailbone.

✳ *Hold for 10 breaths.*

▷ *Release, return to the Child Pose and rest.*

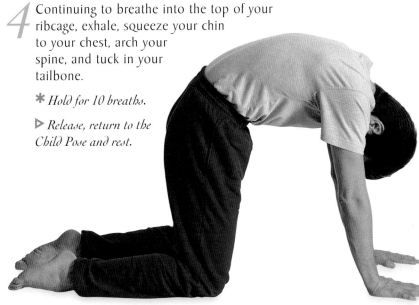

BEGINNER'S PROGRAM

Yoga contains no element of competition so it can be practiced by anyone, of any age.
If you are a newcomer to yoga you should follow the beginner's program, which has
been designed to introduce you to the yoga poses or asanas *as safely as possible.*

You can begin to practice yoga regardless of your age or current physical condition. This book is intended as an introduction to the practice of hatha yoga and contains a series of postures that have been devised to suit a wide range of abilities and expertise.

GETTING STARTED Always start your yoga session with a limbering session (pages 12–15) and finish with at least five minutes of relaxation. Try to get into the habit of practicing the Complete Yoga Breath (pages 10–11) before you begin, to remind yourself to breathe properly throughout your workout, and at the end to help you relax your mind and body.

As a newcomer you should practice the series of poses in the beginner's program three to four times a week. If you wish you can practice everyday. Keep this up for at least two months or until you are thoroughly familiar with the postures. Once you have achieved this you can progress to the more advanced postures found in the intermediate program. Both programs begin with the dynamic Sun Salutation sequence to energize your practice. This is followed by a series of standing, seated, lying, and inverted postures.

Each program includes the six fundamental aspects of a well-balanced yoga routine: forward bends, backward bends, side stretches, spinal twists, balances, and inversions. General information about each posture is given on the upper page, with a complete step-by-step guide to performing the posture on the lower page. Stand the book up on a table at eye level so you can consult it with ease during your practice. The beginner's program should take about one hour to perform.

PRACTICE MAKES PERFECT As a beginner it is especially important that you do not skip any of the poses and that you perform them in the order in which they appear in the book.

The sequence of postures has been specially devised to ensure that the poses complement each other and every part of the body is given a thorough workout. If you find any of the postures too difficult, perform the suggested modifications.

If you can't perform the complete extension of a posture, don't worry: even when you can only manage a movement of a few inches the posture will still prove beneficial. Regular practice of each posture in the beginner's program will ensure steady progress and is the best way to achieve effective and lasting results.

Accompanying the step-by-step instructions for performing and maintaining each posture are the instructions for your breathing. Follow these directions closely, as correct control of the breath helps you to perform many of the postures smoothly and gracefully, especially the dynamic sequences or cycles of postures. When no specific breathing instructions are given, you should simply breathe normally.

ENHANCE YOUR WELL-BEING Yoga has many mental and physical benefits and the chief remedial effects of each *asana* are detailed in the text accompanying the step-by-step pages. These include soothing muscular aches and pains, realigning bad posture, relieving stress, and alleviating long-term conditions

such as asthma, sciatica, and scoliosis. You should notice the positive effects of your posture practice within just a few weeks of starting regular sessions. However, yoga should not be used as a substitute for proper medical attention. If you do have a medical condition such as high blood pressure or a back injury, or if you are pregnant, consult your doctor before beginning a yoga program. Cautions appear on the first page of each posture and you should make sure that you read them thoroughly before you begin.

ADDITIONAL INSTRUCTION *Yoga for Beginners* allows you to learn yoga at your own pace and in the comfort of your own home. However, your practice can be enhanced by joining a yoga class where you will be supervised by a properly qualified teacher. He or she can correct your posture, provide encouragement, and guide your practice. Both the programs in this book may be used as a supplement to supervised lessons or as part of your self-practice.

17

ADJUSTING POSTURE
The supervision of a qualified yoga teacher can help you develop good posture and correct technique, which you will then be able to carry into your individual practice.

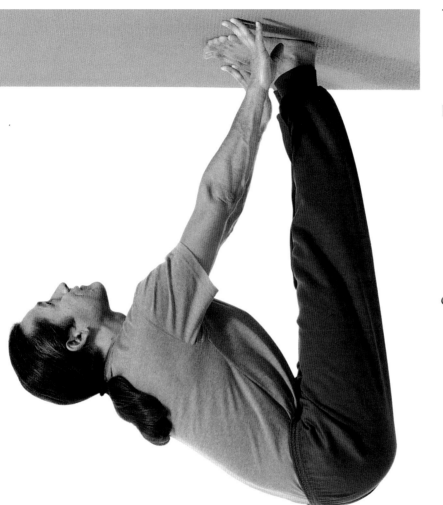

Tadasana to Uttanasana

Mountain Pose to Standing Forward Bend

This dynamic sequence is made up of two important basic poses or *asanas*—the Mountain Pose and the Standing Forward Bend. These two fundamental postures make up the first part of the classic yoga Sun Salutation (see page 50) and are an invigorating way to begin your practice.

Tadasana means "mountain pose" and is the basic standing posture. It allows you to stand firm and tall and helps to realign your body to reduce stiffness. It also supports the spine and holds the internal organs in their healthiest positions.

Uttanasana literally means "intense stretch" and is a wonderfully beneficial posture. It restores elasticity to the spine and legs, improves the circulation of blood to the upper body and brain to relieve depression, and tones the liver, spleen, kidneys, and reproductive organs to help alleviate digestive and menstrual problems.

18

ENCOURAGING
FLEXIBILITY
These postures are especially beneficial for beginners as they rejuvenate the nervous system and increase mobility in the spine and hips.

— TAKE CARE —

If you cannot bend forward with your legs straight, bend your knees to release your lower back. As you progress, try to straighten your legs.

Do not tense your shoulders, neck, or upper back and try to fold into the bend from your lower back and hips.

Practice this posture against a wall to release your hips.

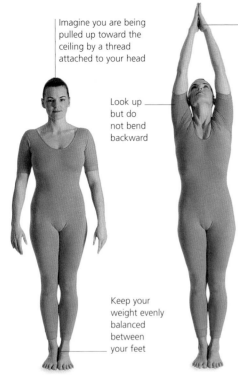

Imagine you are being pulled up toward the ceiling by a thread attached to your head

Your palms should meet as your lungs become fully inflated

Look up but do not bend backward

Keep your weight evenly balanced between your feet

3 Exhale and fold forward from your hips. Bend your knees if necessary. Touch the floor on either side of your toes with your fingertips and place your chin on your knees.

4 Inhale, keeping your fingertips on the floor, and lift your chest. Try to straighten your legs but do not force or strain in the posture.

▷ *Exhale and return to Step 3.*

▷ *Inhale and return to Step 2.*

5 As you exhale, return your hands to your sides. Focus on the balance of weight between your feet and the symmetry of your hips and shoulders.

▷ *Repeat the whole sequence five times without pause.*

Relax your arms by your sides

19

1 Stand with your feet touching. Lift your toes to spread your weight evenly between the balls and heels of your feet. When you are balanced, rest your toes back on the floor and breathe deeply through your nose. This is the Mountain Pose.

2 Inhale and gently stretch your arms away from your sides. Continue to reach up until your palms are pressed together above your head. Look up, focus on your thumbs, and fully extend your body toward the ceiling.

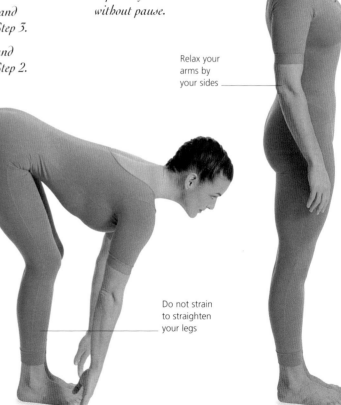

Stretch through to your fingertips as you fold forward

Bring your chin in and down slightly

Do not strain to straighten your legs

Extended Triangle Pose (I)

Utthita Trikonasana

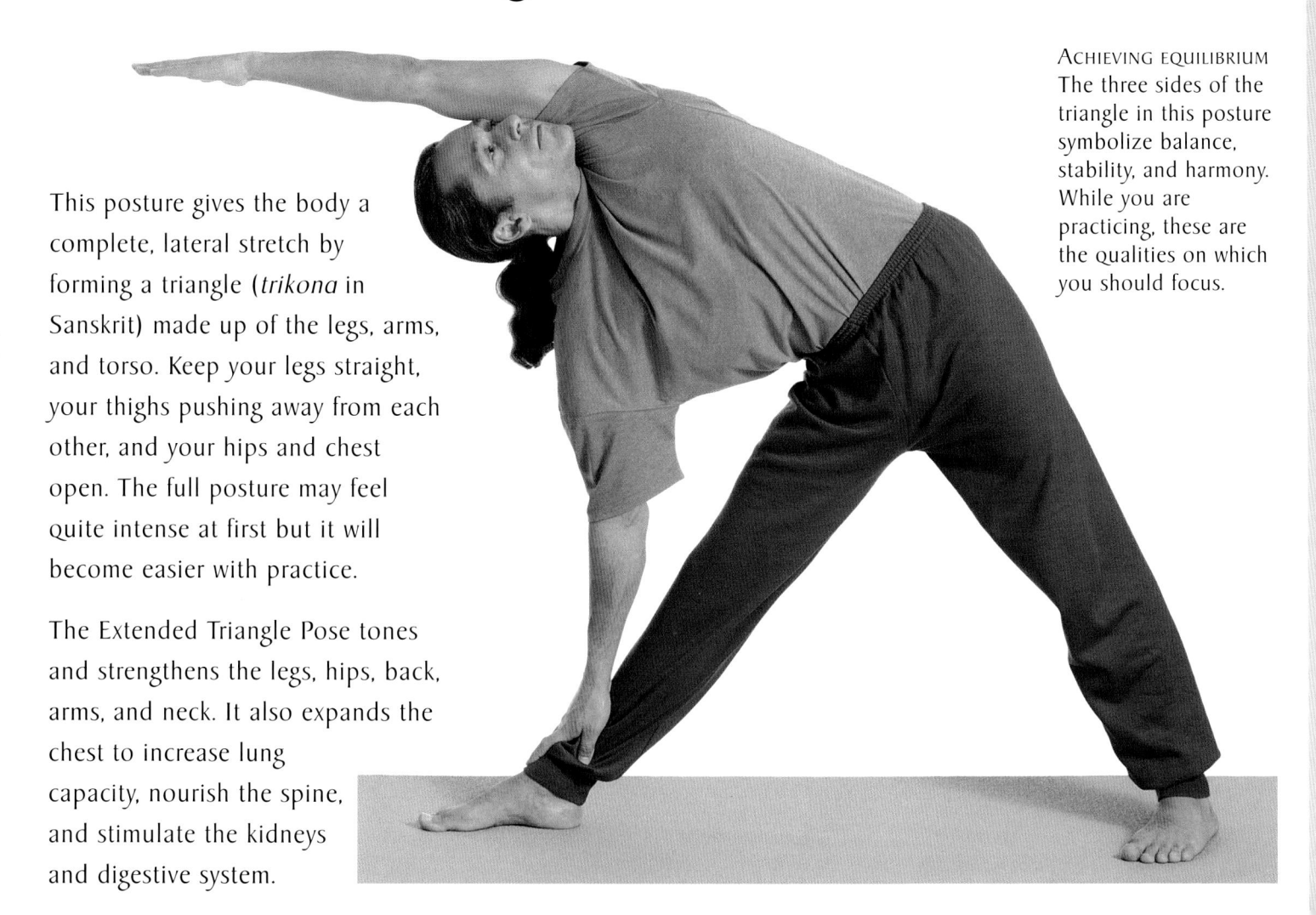

This posture gives the body a complete, lateral stretch by forming a triangle (*trikona* in Sanskrit) made up of the legs, arms, and torso. Keep your legs straight, your thighs pushing away from each other, and your hips and chest open. The full posture may feel quite intense at first but it will become easier with practice.

The Extended Triangle Pose tones and strengthens the legs, hips, back, arms, and neck. It also expands the chest to increase lung capacity, nourish the spine, and stimulate the kidneys and digestive system.

ACHIEVING EQUILIBRIUM
The three sides of the triangle in this posture symbolize balance, stability, and harmony. While you are practicing, these are the qualities on which you should focus.

20

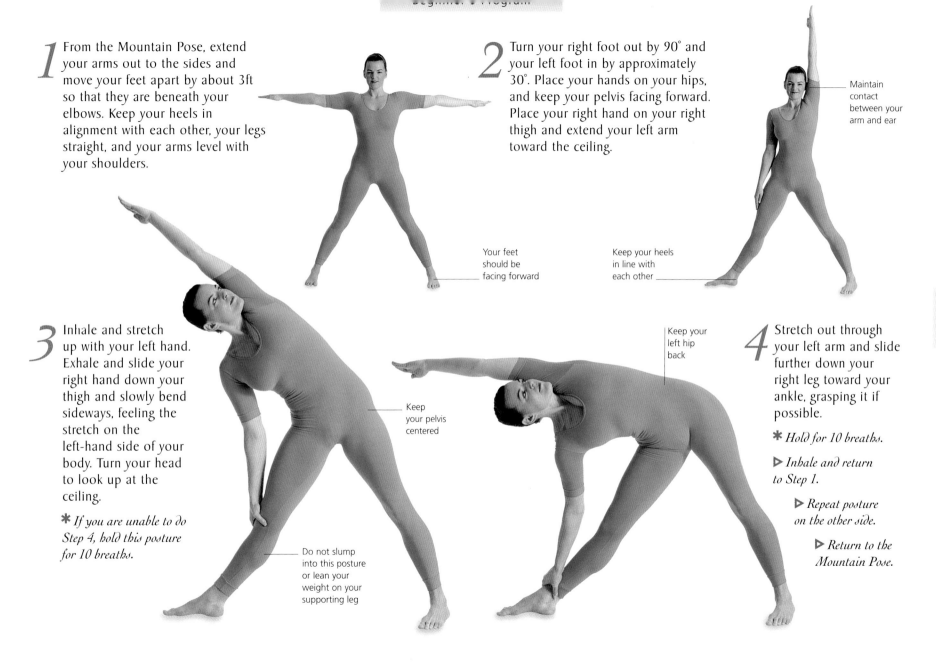

1 From the Mountain Pose, extend your arms out to the sides and move your feet apart by about 3ft so that they are beneath your elbows. Keep your heels in alignment with each other, your legs straight, and your arms level with your shoulders.

2 Turn your right foot out by 90° and your left foot in by approximately 30°. Place your hands on your hips, and keep your pelvis facing forward. Place your right hand on your right thigh and extend your left arm toward the ceiling.

Maintain contact between your arm and ear

Your feet should be facing forward

Keep your heels in line with each other

21

3 Inhale and stretch up with your left hand. Exhale and slide your right hand down your thigh and slowly bend sideways, feeling the stretch on the left-hand side of your body. Turn your head to look up at the ceiling.

✻ *If you are unable to do Step 4, hold this posture for 10 breaths.*

Keep your pelvis centered

Do not slump into this posture or lean your weight on your supporting leg

Keep your left hip back

4 Stretch out through your left arm and slide further down your right leg toward your ankle, grasping it if possible.

✻ *Hold for 10 breaths.*

▷ *Inhale and return to Step 1.*

▷ *Repeat posture on the other side.*

▷ *Return to the Mountain Pose.*

Utthita Parsvakonasana

Extended Side Angle Pose (I)

This posture gets its name from the Sanskrit *parsva* meaning "flank" and *kona* meaning "angle." Its diagonal alignment intensely stretches the entire side of the body, from the shoulder down to the foot. The legs are spread apart in a "warrior" position, so called because it resembles the proud stance of a fighter. This imparts strength and stability to the calves, thighs, ankles, and knees, and also trims the waist and the hips.

The Extended Side Angle Pose improves the function of the lungs and helps respiratory problems by encouraging a deep opening of the chest. The posture also relieves painful conditions affecting the joints, such as sciatica and arthritis, and stimulates peristalsis (the involuntary contractions of the digestive tract), aiding elimination of wastes and cleansing the body of any impurities.

CORRECT ALIGNMENT
This beginner's variation stabilizes the posture by placing the elbow on the knee, which gently leads to the correct alignment of the spine.

▲ *If your hips are stiff, bend your knee a little less and place your hand, rather than your elbow, on your knee. If you have a stiff neck do not look up but face forward instead to avoid placing pressure on the neck.*

— TAKE CARE —

Try to stay as upright as possible, as if sandwiched between two panes of glass. Practice against a wall to help maintain alignment.

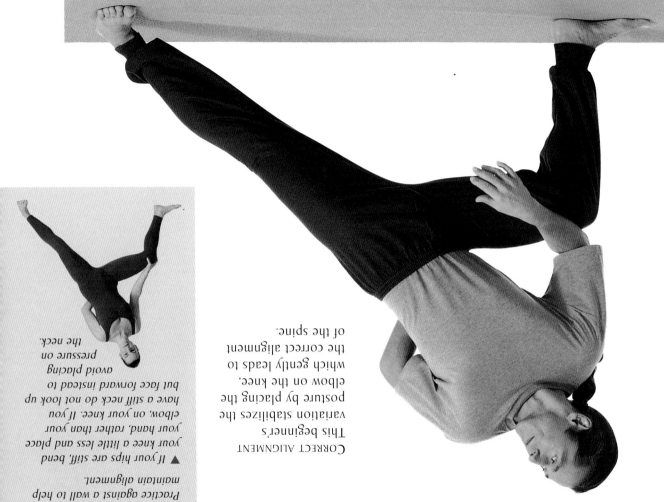

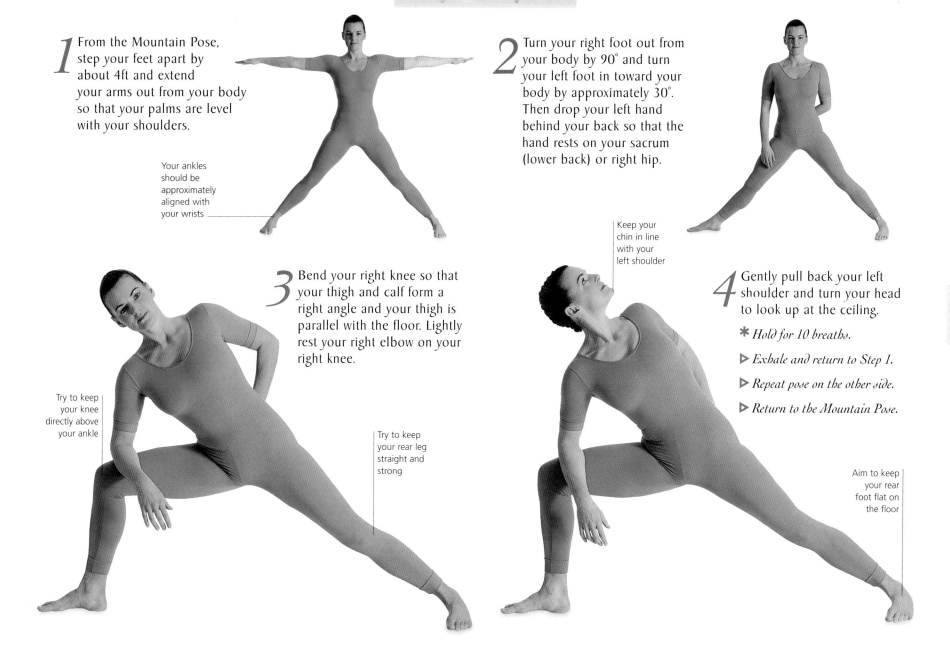

1 From the Mountain Pose, step your feet apart by about 4ft and extend your arms out from your body so that your palms are level with your shoulders.

Your ankles should be approximately aligned with your wrists

2 Turn your right foot out from your body by 90° and turn your left foot in toward your body by approximately 30°. Then drop your left hand behind your back so that the hand rests on your sacrum (lower back) or right hip.

Keep your chin in line with your left shoulder

3 Bend your right knee so that your thigh and calf form a right angle and your thigh is parallel with the floor. Lightly rest your right elbow on your right knee.

Try to keep your knee directly above your ankle

Try to keep your rear leg straight and strong

4 Gently pull back your left shoulder and turn your head to look up at the ceiling.

✳ *Hold for 10 breaths.*

▷ *Exhale and return to Step 1.*

▷ *Repeat pose on the other side.*

▷ *Return to the Mountain Pose.*

Aim to keep your rear foot flat on the floor

23

Padottanasana Extended Foot Pose (I)

The wide positioning of the feet in *Padottanasana*, which means "intense foot stretch," places a thorough, toning extension through the calves and thighs. This helps to loosen the hamstrings and develop the adductor muscles (the inner thigh muscles). The forward bend increases the flow of blood to the torso and head, improving concentration. The deep inversion of the posture invigorates the spine and central nervous system, which helps ease stiffness in the back and hips. It also massages the abdominal organs to soothe the digestive system.

MAINTAINING SYMMETRY
Make sure that your feet are parallel to each other and try to be aware of the alignment of your arms in order to achieve balance and stability in this posture.

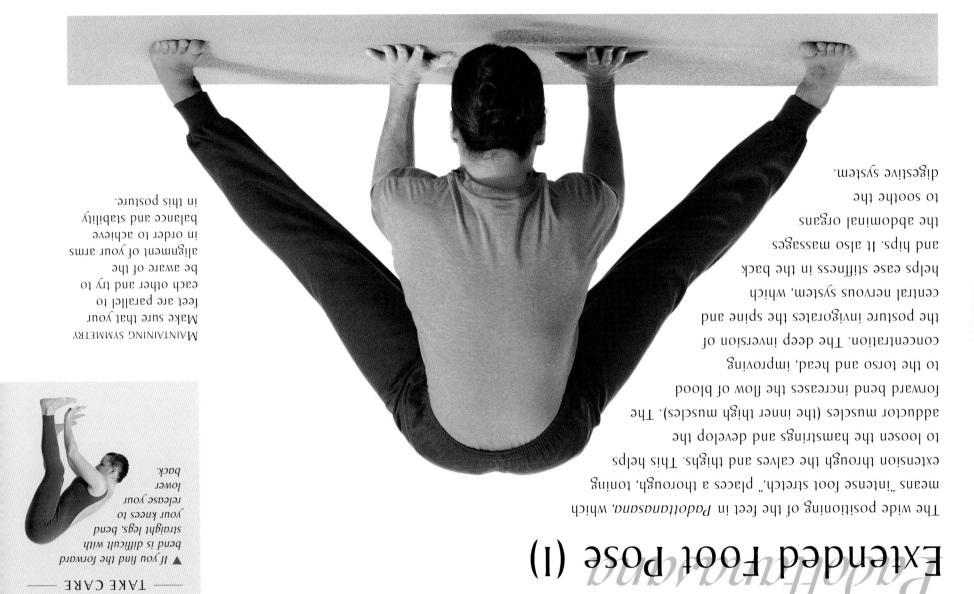

— TAKE CARE —

▲ If you find the forward bend is difficult with straight legs, bend your knees to release your lower back.

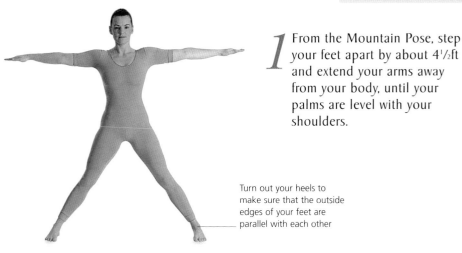

1 From the Mountain Pose, step your feet apart by about 4¹/₂ft and extend your arms away from your body, until your palms are level with your shoulders.

Turn out your heels to make sure that the outside edges of your feet are parallel with each other

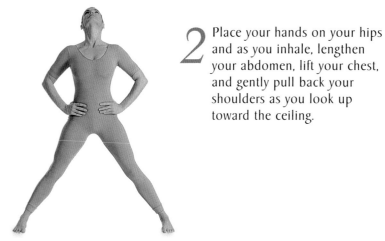

2 Place your hands on your hips and as you inhale, lengthen your abdomen, lift your chest, and gently pull back your shoulders as you look up toward the ceiling.

3 Exhale, fold forward from your hips, and place your fingertips or palms flat on the floor between your feet. Bend your knees slightly if necessary. Inhale, press into the floor, lift your chest, lengthen your abdomen, and look up.

Try to keep your hands shoulder-width apart and your fingertips in line with your toes

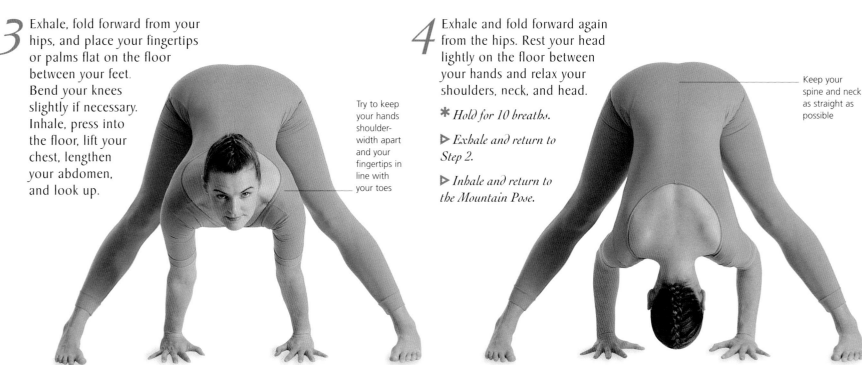

4 Exhale and fold forward again from the hips. Rest your head lightly on the floor between your hands and relax your shoulders, neck, and head.

✱ *Hold for 10 breaths.*

▷ *Exhale and return to Step 2.*

▷ *Inhale and return to the Mountain Pose.*

Keep your spine and neck as straight as possible

Tree Pose (I)

Vrksasana

It is important to attain perfect equilibrium in the Mountain Pose, which is the foundation standing posture, before attempting the more difficult balance of the Tree Pose. Focus on maintaining stability as you lift your foot and transfer your weight onto your supporting leg. As a beginner, you may find it easier to begin the posture with your feet hip-width apart rather than proceeding from the Mountain Pose, with your feet together.

You should aim for tree-like, rooted strength and stability in this posture, which demands both physical poise and concentrated mental focus to master. Although physically simple, the Tree Pose requires highly developed powers of concentration to perform because an unbalanced mind will be reflected in disturbed physical equilibrium. Practice *drushte*—steadily gazing at a fixed point—while performing the posture, to help you maintain both physical balance and mental calm. The movement of body weight onto one foot encourages an erect spine, deepens and tones the chest, and improves the efficiency of the central nervous system. It also tones the legs, limbers the hips, and strengthens the ankles. Most importantly, the Tree Pose encourages a heightened awareness of the body and is thus a good *asana* to perform to improve your general posture and stance.

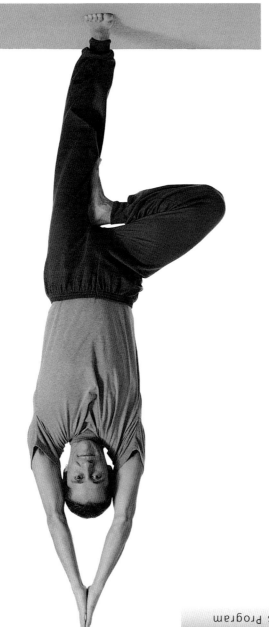

PHYSICAL AWARENESS
It takes practice to develop the necessary sense of balance. However, you will eventually be able to perform the posture with your eyes closed.

— TAKE CARE —

If you have difficulty balancing, use a wall for support.

If your legs and hips are very tight, gently swing your legs and shake out your feet to relax them before and after performing the posture.

If your hips are tight place your raised foot lower down your leg to avoid discomfort.

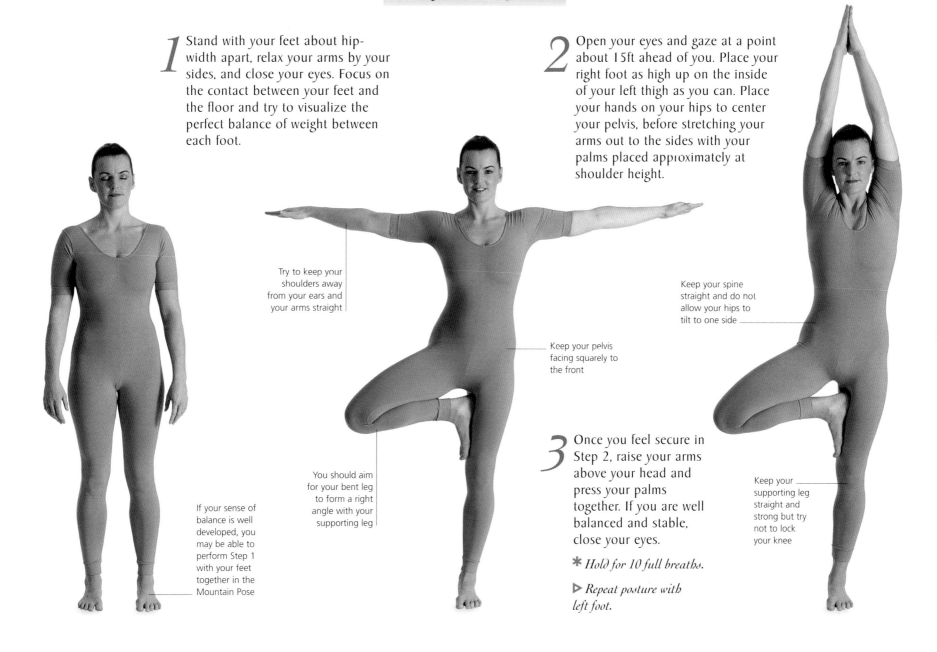

1 Stand with your feet about hip-width apart, relax your arms by your sides, and close your eyes. Focus on the contact between your feet and the floor and try to visualize the perfect balance of weight between each foot.

2 Open your eyes and gaze at a point about 15ft ahead of you. Place your right foot as high up on the inside of your left thigh as you can. Place your hands on your hips to center your pelvis, before stretching your arms out to the sides with your palms placed approximately at shoulder height.

Try to keep your shoulders away from your ears and your arms straight

Keep your spine straight and do not allow your hips to tilt to one side

Keep your pelvis facing squarely to the front

3 Once you feel secure in Step 2, raise your arms above your head and press your palms together. If you are well balanced and stable, close your eyes.

* *Hold for 10 full breaths.*

▷ *Repeat posture with left foot.*

You should aim for your bent leg to form a right angle with your supporting leg

If your sense of balance is well developed, you may be able to perform Step 1 with your feet together in the Mountain Pose

Keep your supporting leg straight and strong but try not to lock your knee

Staff Pose

Dandasana

The sequence of standing *asanas* that you have now performed strengthens and aligns your body in preparation for the more intense twists and extensions that you will encounter in the following set of seated postures.

Danda means "staff" or "rod" and the straight back and limbs of the Staff Pose create the ideal posture in which to perform the seated forward bends. It is important to properly align your body by practicing this foundation posture before moving on to more rigorous seated bends and twists. In the Staff Pose, your spine should be held straight and erect, and your legs should be extended out to the front with your feet flexed. This puts a gentle stretch through the back of the legs and hamstrings to prepare you for the more intense physical work of the seated postures that follow.

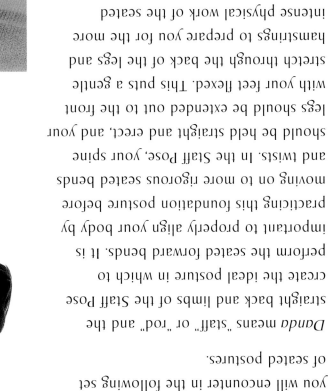

28

PREPARATORY POSTURE
Always practice the Staff Pose before performing any of the more complex seated postures in order to align your body correctly.

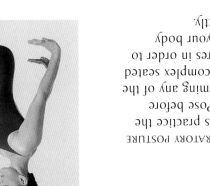

▲ *To encourage the straightening of the spine, place your hands behind you with your fingertips pointing inward. Lift your chest and open your shoulders.*

— TAKE CARE —

Make sure that you are sitting to the front of your sitting bones by lifting your buttocks away behind you or "walking" forward a few inches on your bottom.

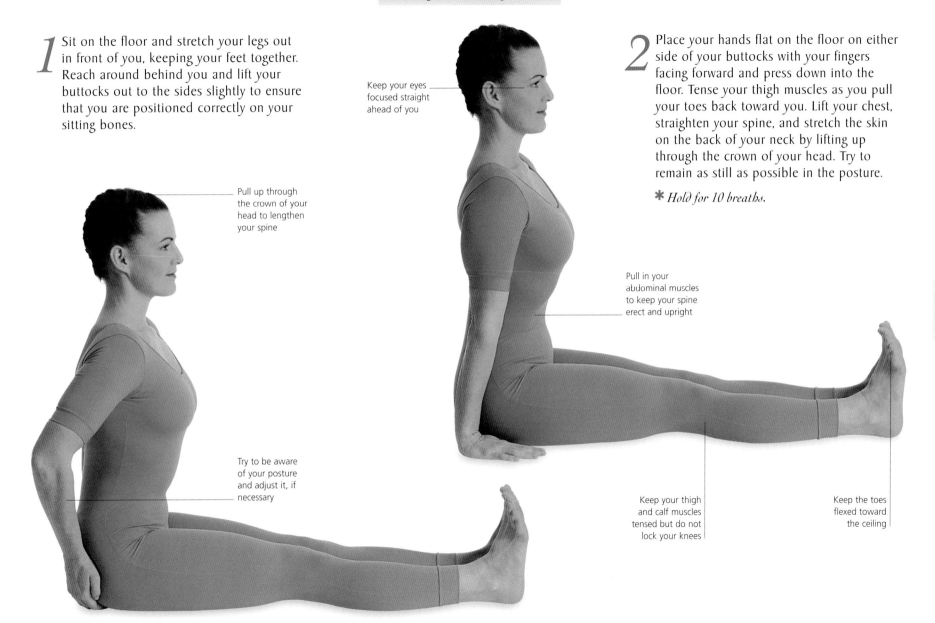

1 Sit on the floor and stretch your legs out in front of you, keeping your feet together. Reach around behind you and lift your buttocks out to the sides slightly to ensure that you are positioned correctly on your sitting bones.

Pull up through the crown of your head to lengthen your spine

Try to be aware of your posture and adjust it, if necessary

Keep your eyes focused straight ahead of you

2 Place your hands flat on the floor on either side of your buttocks with your fingers facing forward and press down into the floor. Tense your thigh muscles as you pull your toes back toward you. Lift your chest, straighten your spine, and stretch the skin on the back of your neck by lifting up through the crown of your head. Try to remain as still as possible in the posture.

✳ *Hold for 10 breaths.*

Pull in your abdominal muscles to keep your spine erect and upright

Keep your thigh and calf muscles tensed but do not lock your knees

Keep the toes flexed toward the ceiling

Seated Forward Bend

Paschimottanasana

Paschima literally translates from Sanskrit as "west," which in the yogic tradition refers to the back of the body, from the head to the heels. Thus *Paschimottanasana* literally means "extending" or "stretching the west" and in this posture the whole of the rear aspect of the body is given an intense stretch. This awakens the spine and central nervous system, stimulating the nerve centers in the lumbar area (the base of the spine), invigorating the brain, stretching the hamstrings and making the loins supple. Internally, this posture stimulates the digestive system, calms the activity of the kidneys, massages the heart, and stimulates the reproductive organs.

As the back of the body is traditionally associated with the west, so the front of the body from the face to the toes is considered to be the eastern aspect, the crown of the head is considered to be the north, and the soles and heels are thought to make up the southern aspect.

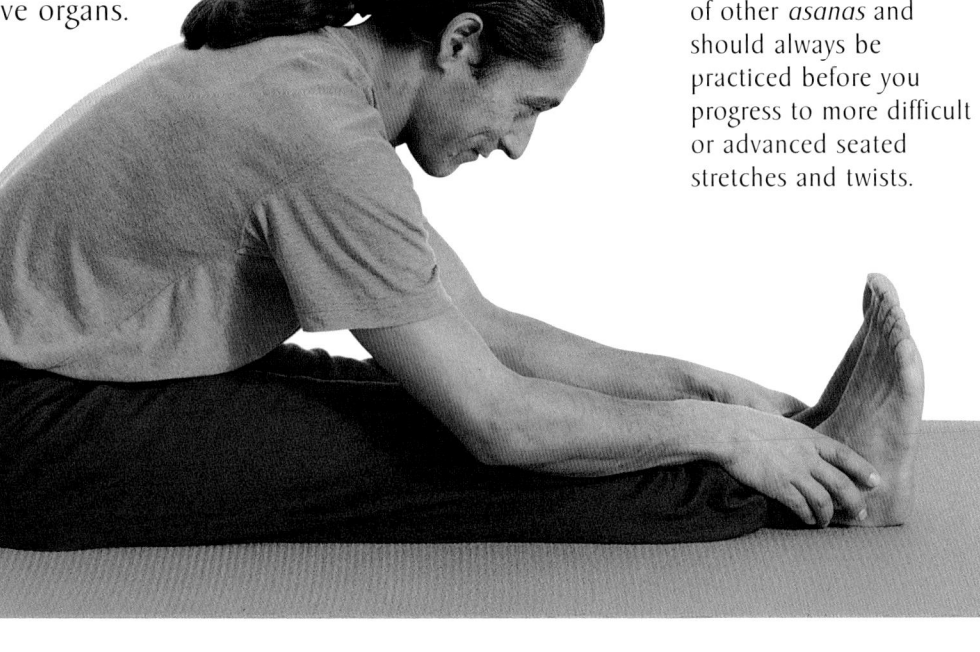

PRINCIPAL FORWARD BEND
This posture is the foundation of a number of other *asanas* and should always be practiced before you progress to more difficult or advanced seated stretches and twists.

30

— TAKE CARE —

Do not worry about how far you can stretch at first. Concentrate instead on your breathing and releasing into the posture smoothly, without forcing or straining your body.

▼ *If your back feels very stiff, bend your knees slightly and link your arms beneath them. Hugging your knees in this way helps to bend the lower back and avoids bowing the upper body.*

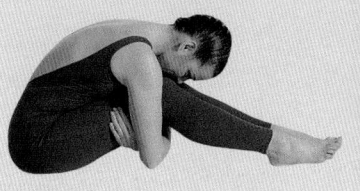

▼ *Alternatively, you may support the forward bend by placing a cushion between your torso and legs or practice by sitting in a chair, bending forward, and dropping your hands to the floor as you do so.*

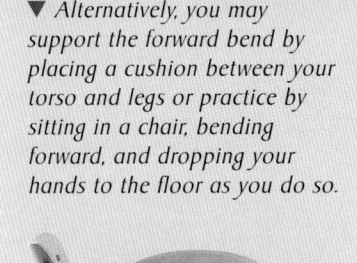

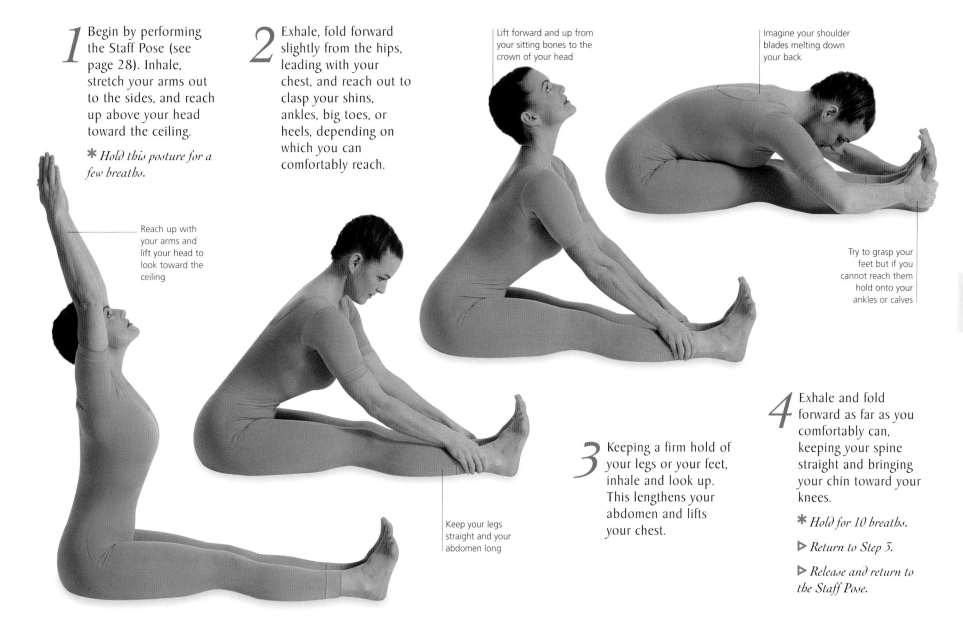

1 Begin by performing the Staff Pose (see page 28). Inhale, stretch your arms out to the sides, and reach up above your head toward the ceiling.

✳ *Hold this posture for a few breaths.*

Reach up with your arms and lift your head to look toward the ceiling

2 Exhale, fold forward slightly from the hips, leading with your chest, and reach out to clasp your shins, ankles, big toes, or heels, depending on which you can comfortably reach.

Lift forward and up from your sitting bones to the crown of your head

Imagine your shoulder blades melting down your back

Try to grasp your feet but if you cannot reach them hold onto your ankles or calves

31

Keep your legs straight and your abdomen long

3 Keeping a firm hold of your legs or your feet, inhale and look up. This lengthens your abdomen and lifts your chest.

4 Exhale and fold forward as far as you comfortably can, keeping your spine straight and bringing your chin toward your knees.

✳ *Hold for 10 breaths.*

▷ *Return to Step 3.*

▷ *Release and return to the Staff Pose.*

One Leg Seated Forward Bend

Janu Sirsasana

Literally translated from Sanskrit as the "head to knee pose," this posture differs from the previous one by directing the forward bend of the body over one knee only. Concentrate on maintaining alignment between your head and the knee of your outstretched leg, as this heightens your awareness of your general posture. As you bend forward, the weight of your torso intensifies the stretch in the straight leg. This loosens the hamstrings in both legs and encourages flexibility in the hips and spine, making it ideal if you have a sedentary lifestyle.

The One Leg Seated Forward Bend has a number of internal benefits: it improves the function of the abdominal organs, aids digestion, and is particularly helpful for men suffering from an enlarged prostate. It can also help reduce the temperature of a mild fever.

32

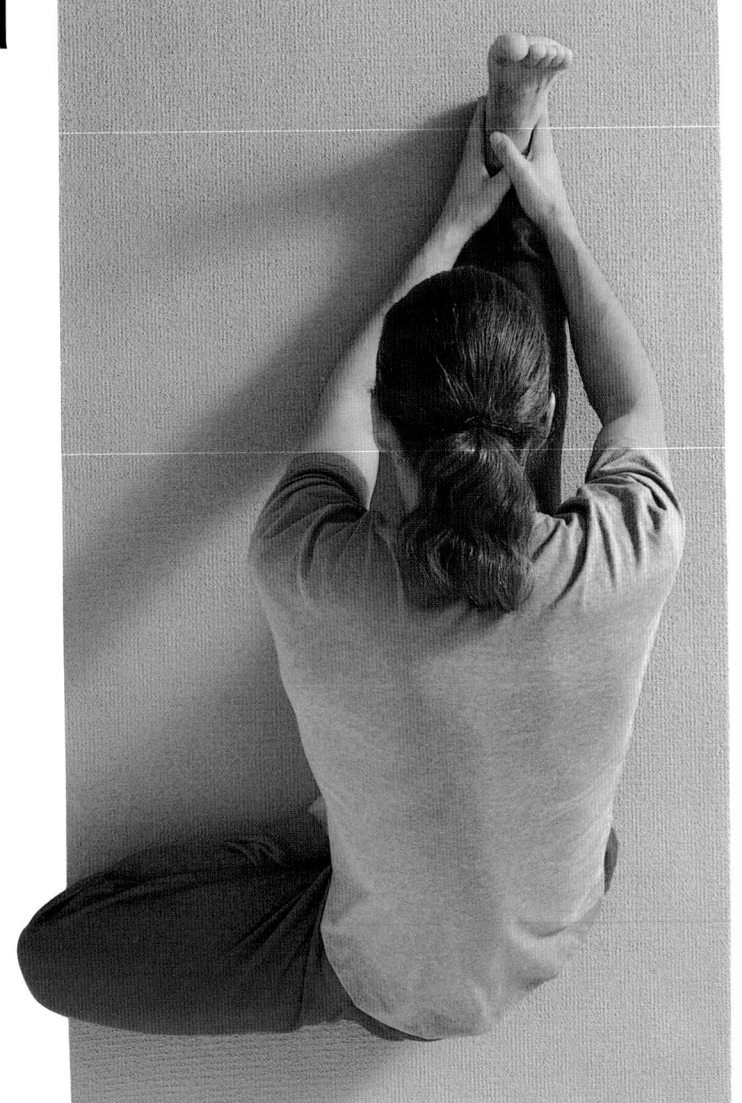

TAKE CARE

Try to direct your torso over your extended leg as you lean forward.

Do not force the pose; simply breathe and release into it.

Lengthen forward from the hips and keep your spine as straight as possible to achieve the maximum benefit from this posture.

GENTLE PROGRESS
Do not worry about the depth of the bend at first. Instead concentrate on maintaining your alignment and the 90° angle of your legs.

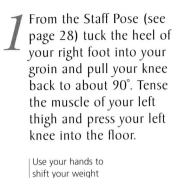

1 From the Staff Pose (see page 28) tuck the heel of your right foot into your groin and pull your knee back to about 90°. Tense the muscle of your left thigh and press your left knee into the floor.

Use your hands to shift your weight forward onto your sitting bones

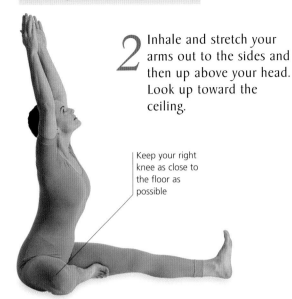

2 Inhale and stretch your arms out to the sides and then up above your head. Look up toward the ceiling.

Keep your right knee as close to the floor as possible

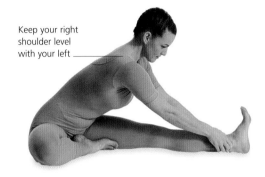

3 As you exhale, fold forward from the hips, stretching through to your fingertips, and grip your shin, ankle, or heel.

Keep your right shoulder level with your left

33

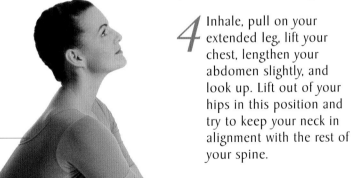

Keep your spine as straight as possible to lengthen your torso

4 Inhale, pull on your extended leg, lift your chest, lengthen your abdomen slightly, and look up. Lift out of your hips in this position and try to keep your neck in alignment with the rest of your spine.

5 Exhale, lengthen forward, and bring your chin toward your left knee. Come down only as far as is comfortable and do not force the posture.

✽ *Hold for 10 breaths.*

▷ *Return to Step 4.*

▷ *Exhale, release posture, and repeat on the other side.*

Extend into the posture from your hips, leading with your chest rather than your head

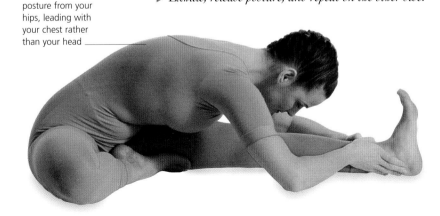

Kneeling Back Bend Cycle

Vajrasana

This sequence is a variation of *Vajrasana*, the "Thunderbolt Pose," and is intended to flow smoothly using *vinyasa* or the "synchronization of breath and movement." This dynamic cycle of bends limbers and awakens the spine and soothes backache.

The combination of forward and backward bends strengthens the spine and encourages flexibility. *Darnikasana*, the "Child Pose," gives a gentle stretch to the spine, hips, and shoulders. Rolling into the Raised Child Pose from this position stimulates blood flow to the face and brain and stretches the neck and lower back, helping to relieve headaches caused by muscular tension. Finally, arching the spine into a back bend opens the chest and encourages deep breathing. The cycle is particularly good for counteracting the physical effects of a sedentary lifestyle.

34

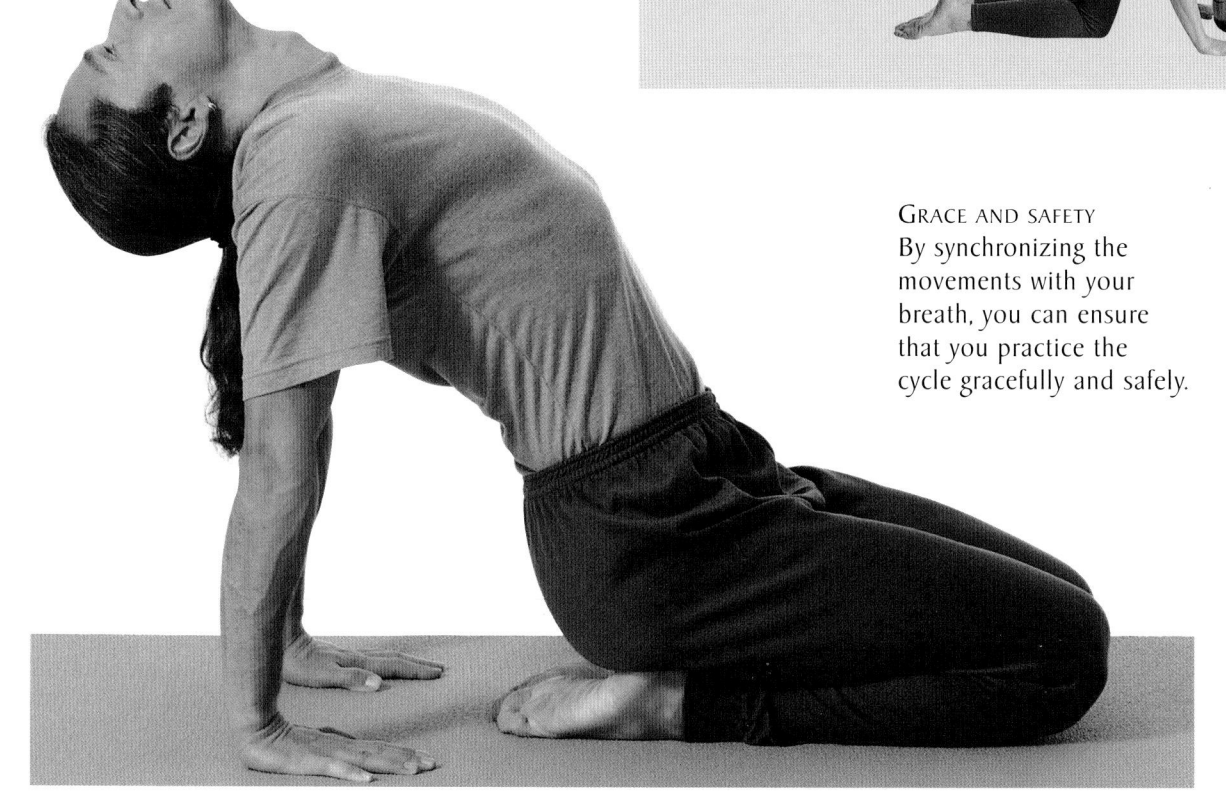

TAKE CARE

Keep your chin tucked into your chest as you arch into the back bend rather than dropping your head back if your neck is at all stiff.

Before you start, you may wish to gently roll your head from side to side and raise and lower your shoulders to warm up your neck.

▼ *If you have a very stiff neck, you could support your head with your hands in the Raised Child Pose.*

GRACE AND SAFETY
By synchronizing the movements with your breath, you can ensure that you practice the cycle gracefully and safely.

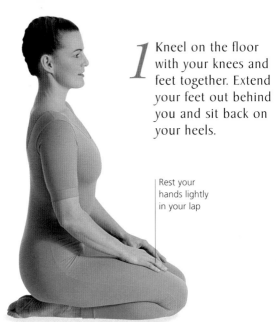

1 Kneel on the floor with your knees and feet together. Extend your feet out behind you and sit back on your heels.

Rest your hands lightly in your lap

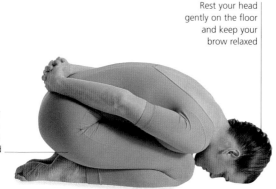

2 Take your arms behind you and interlock your fingers behind your back. Inhale, look up, and arch your spine.

Keep your hands clasped behind you as you open your shoulders and chest

3 Exhale, fold forward, and bring your forehead toward the floor in front of your knees. This is a variation of the Child Pose.

Rest your head gently on the floor and keep your brow relaxed

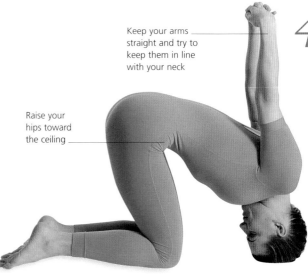

Ensure that your buttocks remain on your heels as you fold forward

Keep your arms straight and try to keep them in line with your neck

Raise your hips toward the ceiling

4 As you inhale, lift your hips and gently roll onto the crown of your head, raising your clasped hands to the ceiling as you do so. This is the Raised Child Pose.

✱ *Hold for 5 breaths.*

▷ *Exhale, return to the Child Pose and rest.*

▷ *Return to Step 1.*

Imagine the center of your breastbone being pulled toward the ceiling

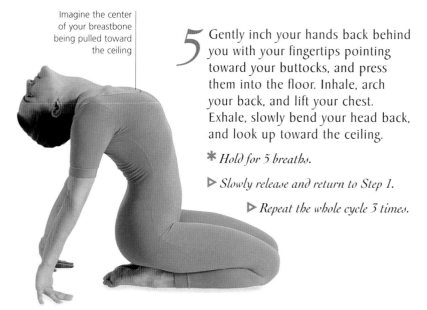

5 Gently inch your hands back behind you with your fingertips pointing toward your buttocks, and press them into the floor. Inhale, arch your back, and lift your chest. Exhale, slowly bend your head back, and look up toward the ceiling.

✱ *Hold for 5 breaths.*

▷ *Slowly release and return to Step 1.*

▷ *Repeat the whole cycle 3 times.*

Seated Spinal Twist (I)

Ardha Matsyendrasana

This posture is named after the sage Matsyendra, one of the first masters of hatha yoga. It provides a rotation of the spine that nourishes and realigns the vertebrae in the upper body and neck. The Seated Spinal Twist also strengthens the neck muscles, opens the shoulders, chest, and hips, corrects scoliosis (curvature of the spine), and helps prevent rheumatic pain and neuralgia.

The twisting movement has a squeezing and massaging effect that preserves the kidneys, tones the adrenal glands, and stimulates the thyroid. It also encourages peristalsis (involuntary contractions of the abdominal tract) to rid the blood and the digestive system of any impurities.

PROTECTING FLEXIBILITY

This twisting seated posture helps keep the spine flexible and elastic. It also promotes mobility of the hip, knee, and shoulder joints.

It is important to keep the spine straight and the chest lifted. Also, lift yourself up out of your sitting bones and keep your shoulders pulled back and level with each other.

▲ *If you have tight hips or knee problems, try this position sitting in a chair. This is also a good modification to use during your working day to release tension in your back and neck.*

TAKE CARE

Hold the posture for a few breaths, lifting your spine with each inhalation and twisting it gently with each exhalation.

▲ *If you have tight hips, you may prefer to keep your lower leg straight.*

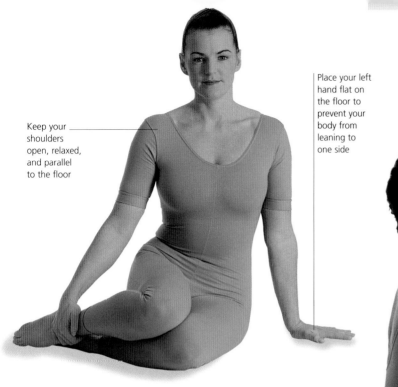

Keep your shoulders open, relaxed, and parallel to the floor

Place your left hand flat on the floor to prevent your body from leaning to one side

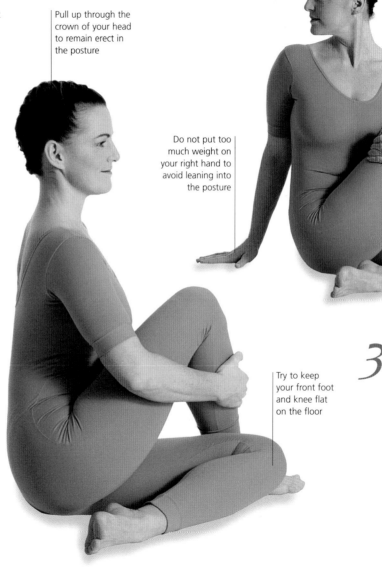

Pull up through the crown of your head to remain erect in the posture

Do not put too much weight on your right hand to avoid leaning into the posture

Try to keep your front foot and knee flat on the floor

Use your left arm to hug your right knee into your chest

1 Kneel on the floor and rest your weight on your left buttock and thigh. Tuck your heels toward your buttocks with your right hand and use your left hand to support yourself.

2 Use your right hand to bring your right foot over your left leg at the knee and place the sole of your foot flat on the floor. Focus on keeping your spine straight.

3 Place your right hand on the floor behind you and with your left hand bring your right knee into your chest. Lift your abdomen as you inhale and as you exhale turn your head to look over your right shoulder.

✳ *Hold for 10 breaths.*

▷ *Repeat on the other side.*

Cobra Pose

Bhujangasana

Bhujanga means "serpent" and in this graceful, back-bending posture, the legs remain on the floor while the trunk of the body is lifted out of the hips and the head is drawn up to form a deep arch—resembling a cobra preparing to strike.

The powerful, toning stretch of the Cobra Pose strengthens the back and fully expands the chest. It corrects misalignments of the spine and, by placing gentle pressure on the abdomen, massages the internal organs to ease menstrual pain and relieve digestive problems. If you are pregnant, you may perform a standing variation of this posture.

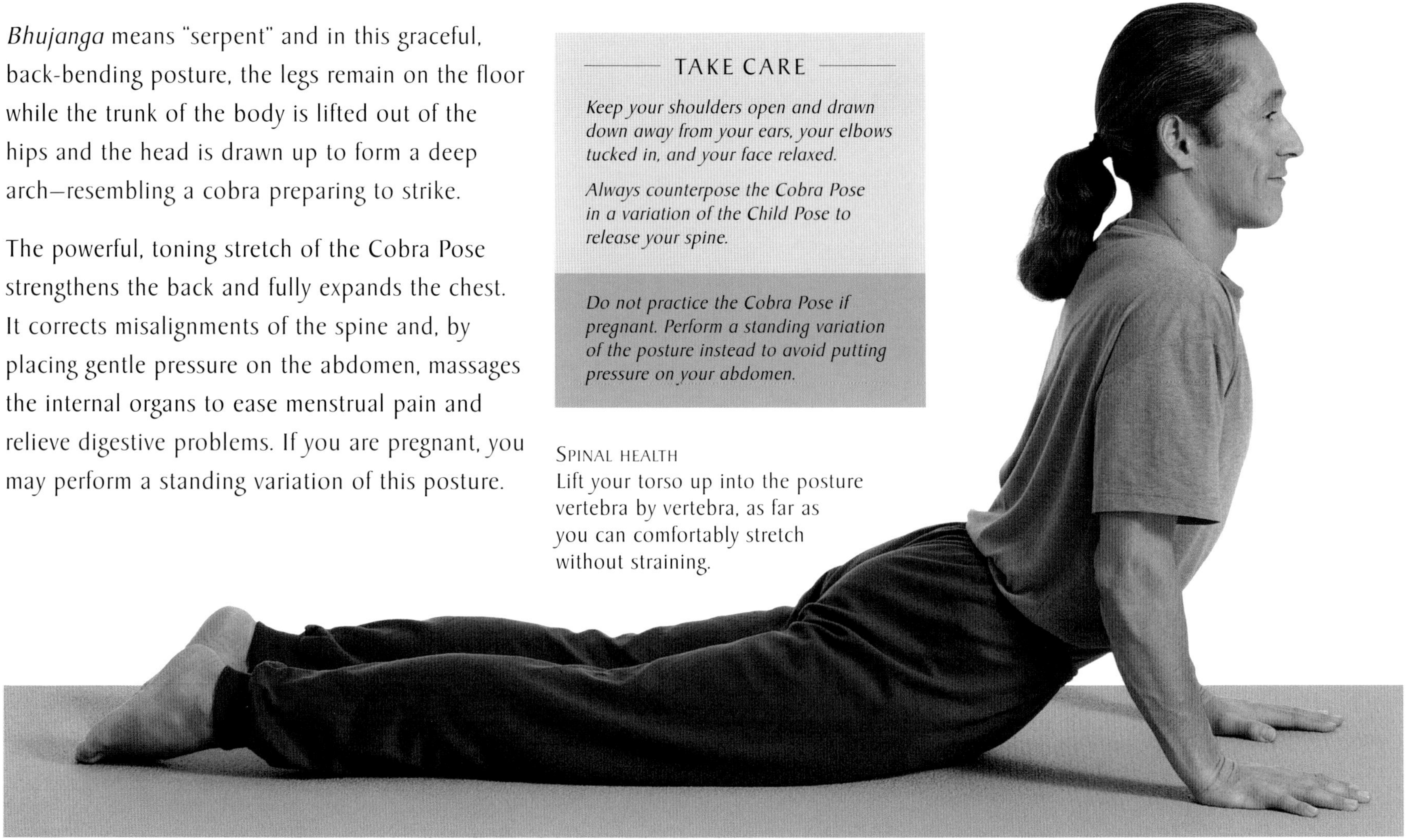

SPINAL HEALTH
Lift your torso up into the posture vertebra by vertebra, as far as you can comfortably stretch without straining.

— TAKE CARE —

Keep your shoulders open and drawn down away from your ears, your elbows tucked in, and your face relaxed.

Always counterpose the Cobra Pose in a variation of the Child Pose to release your spine.

Do not practice the Cobra Pose if pregnant. Perform a standing variation of the posture instead to avoid putting pressure on your abdomen.

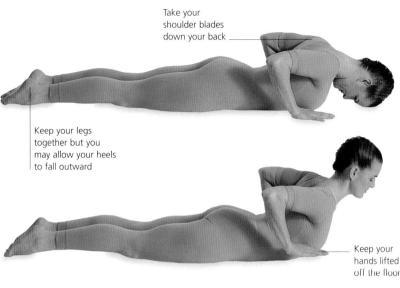

Take your shoulder blades down your back

Keep your legs together but you may allow your heels to fall outward

Keep your hands lifted off the floor

1 Lay down flat on your stomach, place your hands under your shoulders, and rest your forehead on the ground. Your big toes should touch but your heels can fall out to the sides. It is important to keep your feet on the floor at all times.

2 As you inhale, lower the tip of your nose to the floor, followed by your chin. Keep your hands raised slightly so that you are using only your back muscles to lift your torso from the floor.

✱ *Hold for 5 breaths.*

▷ *Exhale and return to Step 1.*

3 Move your hands 1–2 inches back toward your waist and lift your torso again. This time, push gently against the floor with your hands to increase the degree of lift. Keep your head held high and drop your shoulders away from your ears. Open your chest and gently point your toes to increase the stretch in the legs.

✱ *Hold for 5 breaths.*

▷ *Return to Step 1.*

4 When you have completed the posture, push up onto your hands and knees, sit back on your heels, and bend forward at the waist until your forehead rests on the ground. Extend your arms in front of you. This is the Extended Child Pose.

✱ *Rest in this posture for 10 breaths.*

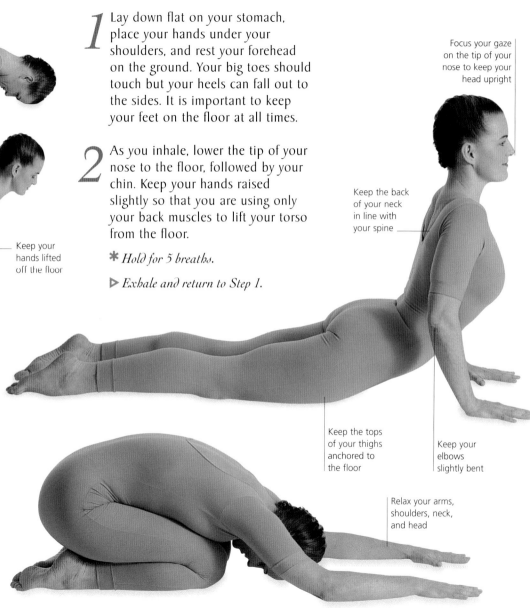

Focus your gaze on the tip of your nose to keep your head upright

Keep the back of your neck in line with your spine

Keep the tops of your thighs anchored to the floor

Keep your elbows slightly bent

Relax your arms, shoulders, neck, and head

Downward Dog Pose

Adho Mukha Svanasana

This posture resembles a dog stretching its front legs down and its hind legs up, hence its name, which literally translates as "down" (*adho*), "facing" (*mukha*), "dog pose" (*svanasana*). It is an energizing posture that relieves physical fatigue and also brings the mental and emotional benefits of inverted postures: increasing blood flow to the trunk of the body, face, and brain, improving concentration, and relieving depression.

The Downward Dog Pose removes stiffness from the joints, particularly in the heels and shoulders, and alleviates arthritis. By lengthening and stretching the calf muscles and hamstrings, flexibility is increased and the legs are shaped and toned. This stretch also promotes speed and agility, making it an excellent posture for runners and other athletes to practice.

REVIVING STRETCH
The stretch in this posture may feel quite intense at first, but brings a wide range of both physical and mental benefits.

TAKE CARE

Make sure that your hands are flat on the floor and your fingers are stretched out and spread apart. Do not twist your wrists.

Lift from your hands, stretching out your torso and hips. Lift your sitting bones as high as possible, relax your neck, and drop your chin toward your chest. If you have trouble straightening your spine, practice with your knees bent.

▼ *Practice your alignment by placing your hands on a wall, shoulder-width apart. Your feet should be hip-width apart and parallel to each other.*

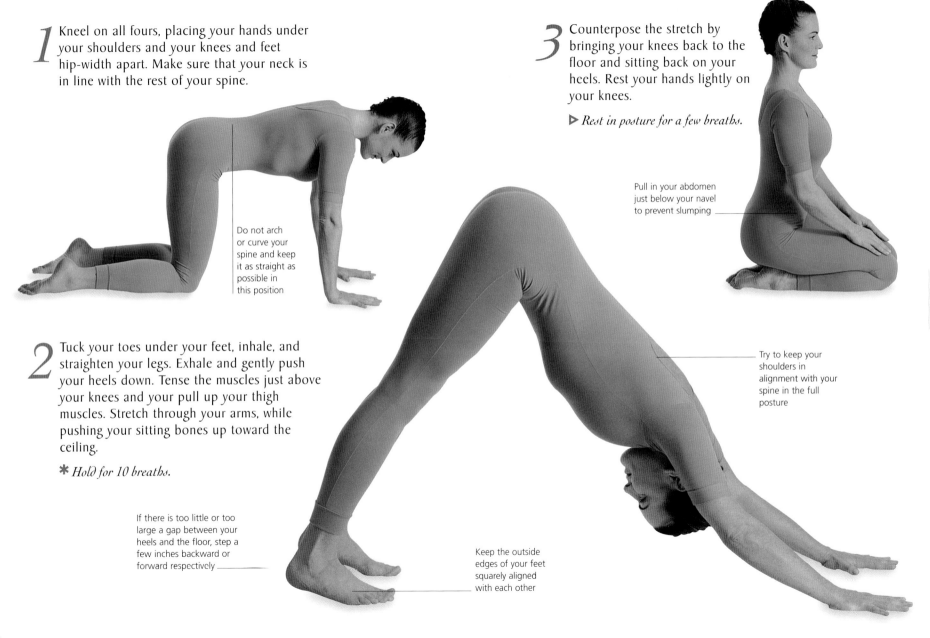

1 Kneel on all fours, placing your hands under your shoulders and your knees and feet hip-width apart. Make sure that your neck is in line with the rest of your spine.

Do not arch or curve your spine and keep it as straight as possible in this position

2 Tuck your toes under your feet, inhale, and straighten your legs. Exhale and gently push your heels down. Tense the muscles just above your knees and your pull up your thigh muscles. Stretch through your arms, while pushing your sitting bones up toward the ceiling.

✳ *Hold for 10 breaths.*

If there is too little or too large a gap between your heels and the floor, step a few inches backward or forward respectively

3 Counterpose the stretch by bringing your knees back to the floor and sitting back on your heels. Rest your hands lightly on your knees.

▶ *Rest in posture for a few breaths.*

Pull in your abdomen just below your navel to prevent slumping

Try to keep your shoulders in alignment with your spine in the full posture

Keep the outside edges of your feet squarely aligned with each other

Pelvic Lift

Urdhva Dhanurasana

Literally translated as the "upward bow pose," *Urdhva Dhanurasana* is so called because it creates a smooth, upward curve of the body that is supported on the shoulders and feet. The Pelvic Lift stretches the front of the body (which is traditionally associated with the east) and is thus a good counterpose to *asanas* that stretch the back or "western" aspect of the body (see the Seated Forward Bend page 30). The chest and abdomen are lifted, which strengthens the abdominal and lower back muscles, and limbers the spine to make it supple (see page 13).

If you find the stretch too intense at first, you may vary the posture to provide more support in the arch of your back, either by placing your hands at your waist or by laying your arms straight along the floor and clasping your hands. This will squeeze your shoulder blades together to open out the front of your chest and strengthen the back of your neck.

42

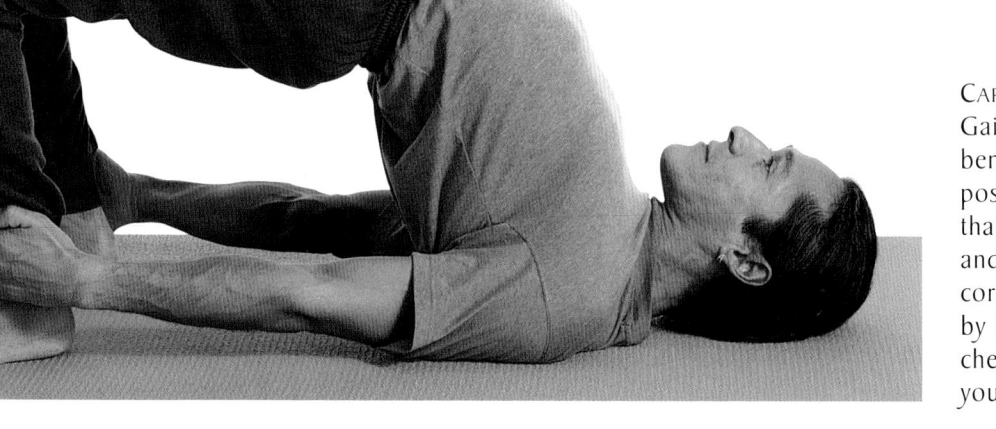

TAKE CARE

Move in and out of the posture slowly and smoothly, synchronizing your movements with deep breathing.

▼ *To develop flexibility safely, lie over a rolled-up blanket or cushions, either while kneeling or on your back with your legs stretched out. First lean back on your elbows, then, when you are comfortable, stretch your arms over your head to stretch your spine. Keep your neck relaxed.*

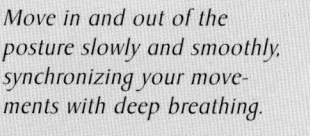

▲ *After performing the Pelvic Lift always counterpose by bringing your knees to your chest to release the sacrum.*

Place your feet parallel to one another. Don't roll onto the outside edges of your feet, but press down through your big toes as you lift up.

CAREFUL POSITIONING
Gain the maximum benefit from the posture by making sure that your feet, legs, and shoulders are correctly aligned and by lifting through your chest as well as from your hips.

1 Lay on your back in the Corpse Pose and step both heels in toward your buttocks. Step your feet hip-width apart and turn your heels out slightly so that your feet are squarely aligned with each other.

Keep your knees no more than hip-width apart

Press your shoulders away from your ears and into the floor

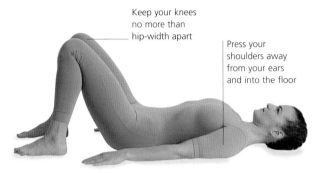

2 Press both hands flat into the floor and, as you inhale, lift your pelvis and arch your back. Press down on the inside edges of your feet and try not to let your knees fall toward each other.

* *Hold for 5 breaths.*

Use your abdominal muscles to lift your body

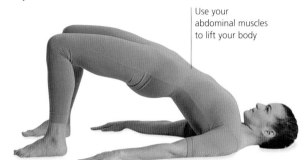

3 As you exhale, lower yourself to the floor, hug your knees to your chest and bring your forehead toward your knees. Gently rock from side-to-side and backward and forward for a few breaths. This counter-posture is the Supine Curl (see page 13).

▷ *Return to Step 1.*

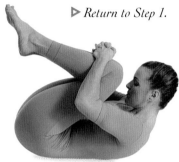

43

Keep your feet flat on the floor throughout the posture

4 Raise your pelvis and interlock your fingers behind your back, keeping your arms straight. In this variation, roll your shoulder blades in toward each other, keeping your hands clasped on the floor.

* *Hold for 5 breaths.*

▷ *Repeat Step 3.*

▷ *Return to Step 1.*

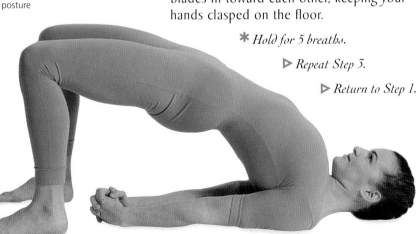

5 Reset your feet as in Step 1, but this time try to reach around and grasp your ankles. As you inhale, lift your pelvis up toward the ceiling in the full extension of the posture. Try to keep your heels on the floor.

* *Hold for 5 breaths.*

▷ *Repeat Step 3.*

▷ *Return to the Corpse Pose.*

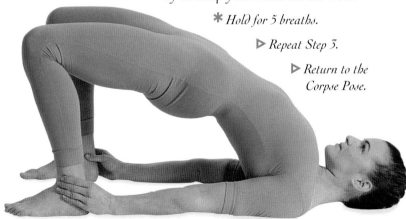

Half Shoulderstand

Ardha Sarvangasana

The name *Sarvangasana* comes from the Sanskrit words for "all limbs" and "whole body." Thus, the full posture is also called the "all-parts pose" and is considered a panacea for common ailments such as colds, headaches, and digestive problems. The posture is also known as the "mother of all *asanas*" because of the rejuvenating effect that it has on the entire body.

The Half Shoulderstand does not require the same degree of balance and control that is needed to practice the full posture (see page 78) or other complex inverted postures. Nonetheless, it provides many of the benefits of the full inversion, increasing the circulation of healthy blood to the heart, chest, and head, calming the mind, and encouraging concentration.

44

CLEANSING BREATH
The restriction of the top of the lungs in this posture activates deep abdominal breathing, which expels toxins and wastes.

TAKE CARE

If you have high blood pressure, practice a variation of the posture by lying with your hips and legs against a wall.

▼ *To enter the posture safely, use a wall for support. Keeping your feet against the wall, bend your knees and lift your hips, using the wall to walk up safely. This is a good variation of the posture to use during pregnancy.*

Do not practice a Half or Full Shoulderstand if you have high blood pressure.

1 Lay on the floor with your arms by your sides. Press your hands flat into the floor and bend your knees in to your chest.

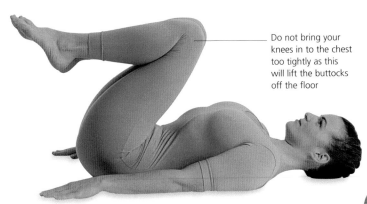

Do not bring your knees in to the chest too tightly as this will lift the buttocks off the floor

2 Straighten your legs up toward the ceiling, keeping your buttocks on the floor. As you inhale, lift your buttocks and swing your legs up but do not attempt to touch your feet to the floor behind your head.

Keep your legs as straight as possible to maintain the stretch in your thighs and calves

45

3 Support your pelvis with your hands and carefully lift your legs 45° from the floor, keeping them as straight as possible. Support your pelvis with your hands, relax your face and keep your throat open and your breathing easy. Do not turn your head in this position.

✱ *Hold for 30 breaths.*

There should be an angle of about 90° between your torso and your legs

4 As you exhale, gently lower your knees toward your forehead, extend your arms and roll down slowly, vertebra by vertebra, bringing your buttocks to rest on your hands.

▷ *Return to the Corpse Pose.*

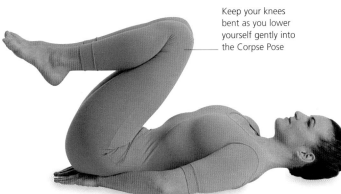

Keep your knees bent as you lower yourself gently into the Corpse Pose

Keep your head on the floor and rest for a few moments before entering the next posture

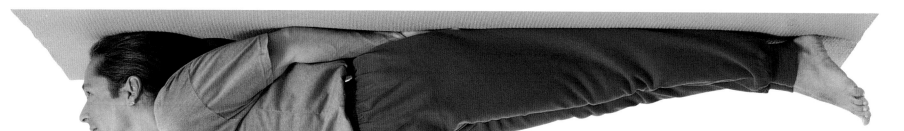

Fish Pose (I)

Matsyasana

This posture is a good counterpose to the Half Shoulderstand because the arching of the back opens the upper chest to reverse the restriction of the shoulders of the previous posture. This opening encourages clavicular, as opposed to abdominal, breathing (see page 10) which tones the upper chest and relieves stiffness and tension in the shoulders and neck.

The Fish Pose contracts the vertebrae in the back of the neck in a further counterpose to the Shoulderstand, which intensely stretches this area. Practicing the two postures together benefits the thyroid (located in the back of the neck) to increase the body's metabolic efficiency and improve energy levels. The thyroid also controls the absorption of calcium, which in turn regulates the contraction of muscles, including the heart, and ensures the strength of bones and teeth. The Fish Pose limbers the pelvic joints and stretches the legs and toes to correct minor postural misalignments.

OPENING THE CHEST
Regular practice of this posture encourages an expansion of the ribcage that improves lung capacity and can help ease respiratory problems such as asthma.

TAKE CARE

When you drop your head back, keep your face and neck completely relaxed. Try to lift your chest as high as possible to fully expand your ribcage and encourage deep breathing.

▲ If you have a stiff neck or other neck problems, keep your head lifted from the floor in the posture. This avoids placing pressure on the head and neck.

1 Lie on the floor with your buttocks resting on the palms of your hands and your elbows as close together as possible beneath you.

Place your hands palms-down on the floor to support your spine and buttocks

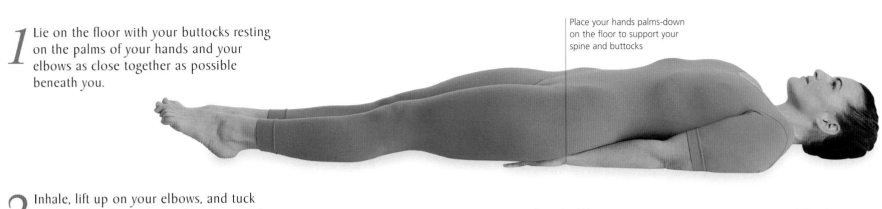

2 Inhale, lift up on your elbows, and tuck your head under to bring the crown of the head gently to the floor. Imagine that the middle of your breastbone is being pulled toward the ceiling by a thread.

 * Hold for 15 breaths.

Keep your legs together and your knees straight and do not allow your feet to fall outward

Your elbows should be tucked in so that they, rather than your head and neck, take your weight

Try to keep your throat open and relaxed to facilitate deep breathing

47

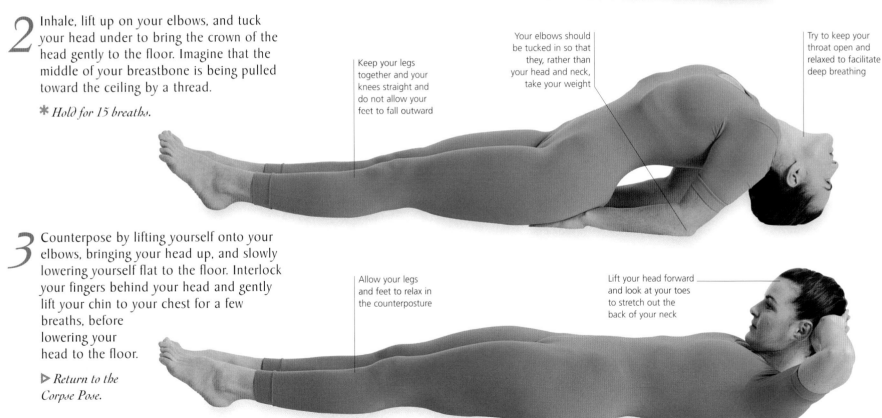

3 Counterpose by lifting yourself onto your elbows, bringing your head up, and slowly lowering yourself flat to the floor. Interlock your fingers behind your head and gently lift your chin to your chest for a few breaths, before lowering your head to the floor.

 ▶ Return to the Corpse Pose.

Allow your legs and feet to relax in the counterposture

Lift your head forward and look at your toes to stretch out the back of your neck

INTERMEDIATE PROGRAM

This series of asanas *should be attempted only once you are familiar with the beginner's program. The intermediate program guides you through the full extensions of the basic postures and introduces some more advanced elements of yoga practice.*

A certain degree of expertise and familiarity is assumed in the intermediate program, both in the general information and in the step-by-step guide to each posture. Therefore, it's important that you are reasonably familiar with the basic postures before you attempt those in this section. However the intermediate program still aims to cater for a range of abilities, so you don't have to be an advanced yoga student to practice the majority of these postures.

FAMILIAR POSES As well as introducing more complex techniques of yoga, this series of *asanas* increases the intensity of some familiar balances, stretches, and extensions. The program begins with a full Sun Salutation—completing the dynamic sequence which first appears in the beginner's program—then moves into a series of individual, static postures.

Remember to limber your body and awaken your spine properly before you begin your yoga practice. As with the beginner's program, make sure you relax properly afterward, incorporating the Complete Yoga Breath (see page 10). More advanced breathing techniques are explored at the end of this program.

When an *asana* in this series is an advanced variation of a basic or foundation posture from the beginner's program, a small, repeat image of the posture will appear on the upper page. This serves to remind you of the standard you should have already reached and helps to demonstrate the progression you will achieve in the intermediate program. Before practicing any of the more advanced seated forward bends in this series (see pages 60-3) be sure to practice the Staff Pose (page 28) and the basic Seated Forward Bend (page 30).

INCREASED FITNESS The intermediate program includes a greater number of dynamic *vinyasa* or breath synchronized sequences of movements. These require both controlled breathing and physical stamina.

You should not expect immediate mastery of these *vinyasa* postures, but if you find them extremely strenuous, spend some more time working through the beginner's program to build up your general fitness.

BE SENSITIVE TO YOUR NEEDS Each student of yoga is an individual, with differing strengths and weaknesses. You may find some of the poses easier to master than others, but if you have difficulty performing a particular posture, do not force your body to achieve the full extension or skip the problematic exercise altogether. Instead, practice the suggested modification or the beginner's variation. If you find that the majority of the postures in this program are too difficult, return to the beginner's series for

a few more weeks until you have built up sufficient strength and flexibility to move on. Continue to observe the cautions, especially if you know you have a particular physical weakness or medical condition.

WORKING WITH A PARTNER You may wish to vary your practice in this program by working with a partner. This can introduce movement into otherwise static poses—deepening and extending the postures—and provide interest and encouragement. If you decide to work with a partner, make sure he or she has practical knowledge of yoga and has reached a similar standard to yourself. An ideal posture to perform together is the variation of the Wide Leg Seated Forward Bend (see page 68), shown below.

49

PARTNER PRACTICE
Performing yoga with a partner deepens your practice and provides you with moral support.

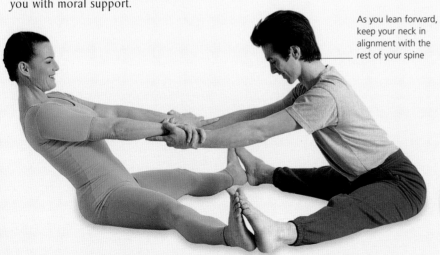

As you lean forward, keep your neck in alignment with the rest of your spine

Bend from your hips in order to keep your back straight

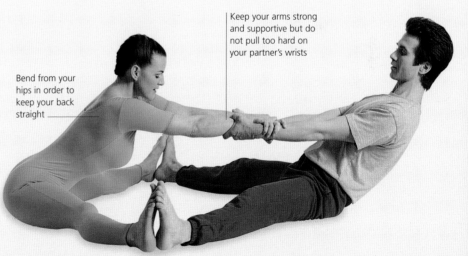

Keep your arms strong and supportive but do not pull too hard on your partner's wrists

Sun Salutation

Surya Namaskar

This invigorating sequence prepares you for the exertions of the day and is traditionally performed before sunrise, hence its name. *Surya Namaskar*, meaning "Salute to the sun." It often begins a yoga session, as it energizes the body and helps you gain flexibility in preparation for individual, static yoga poses.

The Sun Salutation is not a single *asana*, but a dynamic sequence of postures, synchronized with the breathing to flow together smoothly and create *vinyasa*. The fluid movement from one posture to another tones and revitalizes the body, realigning the spine and skeletal system, encouraging deep breathing, and increasing blood flow to all the vital systems of the body. You should already be familiar with some of the postures in the sequence—for example, the Mountain Pose to the Standing Forward Bend (or Half Sun Salutation, see page 18), which makes up the first two movements of this sequence, and the Downward Dog Pose (see page 40). The more advanced *asanas* that appear here as part of the Sun Salutation will be dealt with individually, in greater detail, later in this program. The sequence in which you should perform the postures is demonstrated on the following page; perform them fluidly and without pause before returning to your starting posture to create a complete cycle.

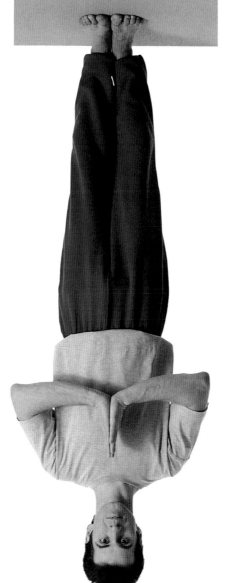

Foundation Postures

Mountain Pose (left)
Standing Forward Bend (right)

PRAYER POSITION
The *Namaskar* hand posture signifies both respectful greeting and prayer in many cultures. It traditionally begins and ends the Sun Salutation sequence.

TAKE CARE

When you roll over your toes into Upward Dog, keep your feet relaxed. If you are uncomfortable, turn your feet back. If this posture places too much pressure on your lower back, keep your thighs on the floor and perform the Cobra Pose (see page 38) instead. If you find holding the Sloping Plank very strenuous, drop your knees to the floor.

50

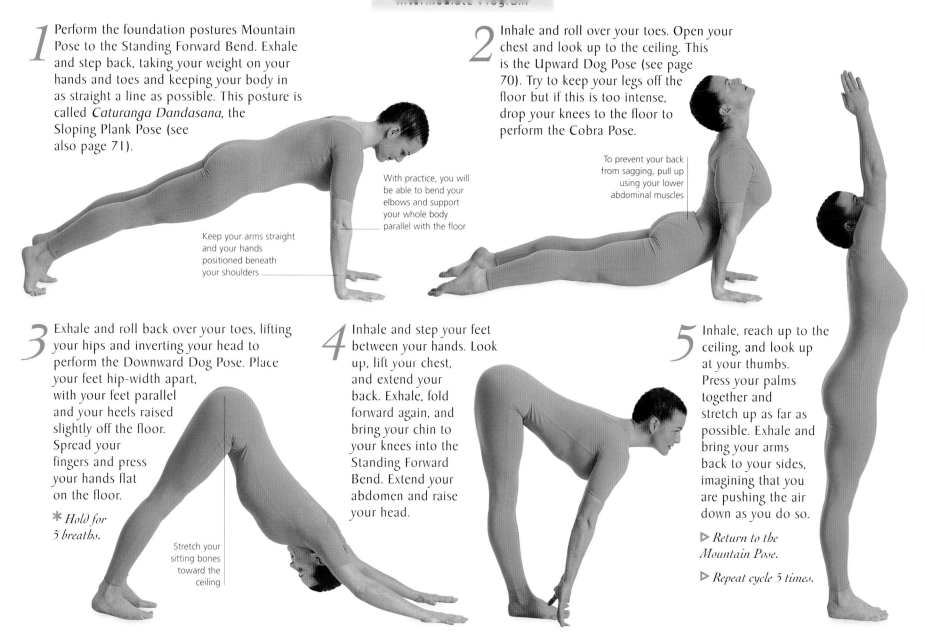

1 Perform the foundation postures Mountain Pose to the Standing Forward Bend. Exhale and step back, taking your weight on your hands and toes and keeping your body in as straight a line as possible. This posture is called *Caturanga Dandasana*, the Sloping Plank Pose (see also page 71).

With practice, you will be able to bend your elbows and support your whole body parallel with the floor

Keep your arms straight and your hands positioned beneath your shoulders

2 Inhale and roll over your toes. Open your chest and look up to the ceiling. This is the Upward Dog Pose (see page 70). Try to keep your legs off the floor but if this is too intense, drop your knees to the floor to perform the Cobra Pose.

To prevent your back from sagging, pull up using your lower abdominal muscles

3 Exhale and roll back over your toes, lifting your hips and inverting your head to perform the Downward Dog Pose. Place your feet hip-width apart, with your feet parallel and your heels raised slightly off the floor. Spread your fingers and press your hands flat on the floor.

✳ *Hold for 5 breaths.*

Stretch your sitting bones toward the ceiling

4 Inhale and step your feet between your hands. Look up, lift your chest, and extend your back. Exhale, fold forward again, and bring your chin to your knees into the Standing Forward Bend. Extend your abdomen and raise your head.

5 Inhale, reach up to the ceiling, and look up at your thumbs. Press your palms together and stretch up as far as possible. Exhale and bring your arms back to your sides, imagining that you are pushing the air down as you do so.

▷ *Return to the Mountain Pose.*

▷ *Repeat cycle 5 times.*

Extended Triangle Pose (II)

The lateral stretch of the beginner's posture (see page 20) is deepened in this program by gripping the ankle or big toe with the right hand, or by placing it flat on the floor behind your foot. A more profound expansion of the chest is encouraged by stretching the other arm up from the shoulder so that it is raised toward the ceiling and forms a vertical line with the lower arm. This posture tones the muscles of the legs to remove stiffness, corrects alignment, and strengthens the spine, hips, and ankles.

Make sure you have mastered the Extended Triangle Pose (I) and can hold it comfortably with stability and balance before attempting the more advanced and intense variation of the posture that is shown in this program.

52

TAKE CARE

Keep your hips open and your legs strong and firm. Pull up just above the knees and through the thigh muscles.

Do not force or strain in this posture. Breathe deeply throughout.

Keep your hips and shoulders against a wall as you stretch to correct your alignment.

HARMONIOUS ALIGNMENT
Try to move through the sequence of steps as fluidly and gracefully as possible, focusing on the symmetry and alignment of the arms, hips, and legs to maintain stability.

Foundation Posture
Extended Triangle (I)

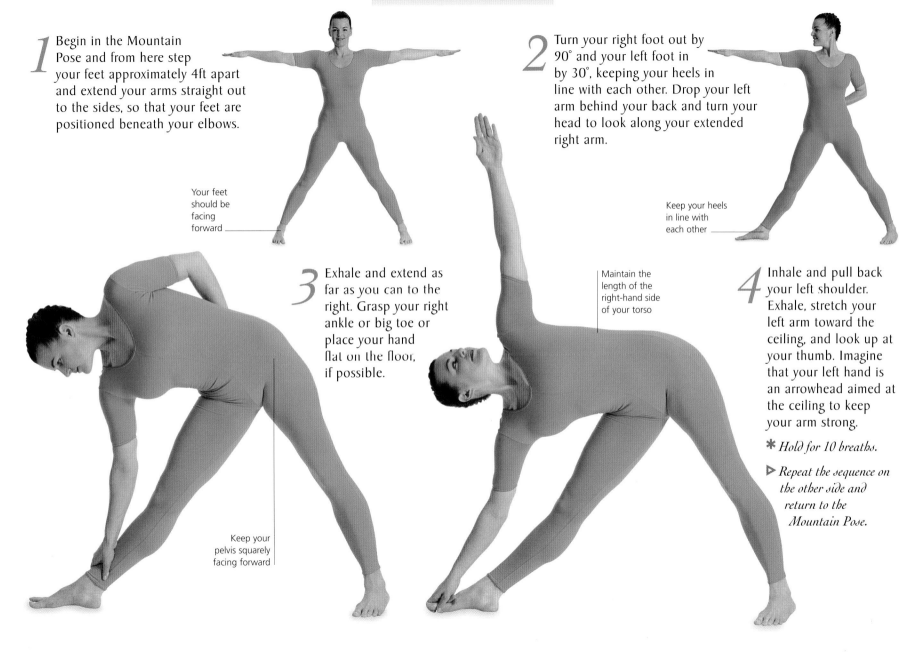

1 Begin in the Mountain Pose and from here step your feet approximately 4ft apart and extend your arms straight out to the sides, so that your feet are positioned beneath your elbows.

Your feet should be facing forward

2 Turn your right foot out by 90° and your left foot in by 30°, keeping your heels in line with each other. Drop your left arm behind your back and turn your head to look along your extended right arm.

Keep your heels in line with each other

3 Exhale and extend as far as you can to the right. Grasp your right ankle or big toe or place your hand flat on the floor, if possible.

Maintain the length of the right-hand side of your torso

Keep your pelvis squarely facing forward

4 Inhale and pull back your left shoulder. Exhale, stretch your left arm toward the ceiling, and look up at your thumb. Imagine that your left hand is an arrowhead aimed at the ceiling to keep your arm strong.

✳ *Hold for 10 breaths.*

▷ *Repeat the sequence on the other side and return to the Mountain Pose.*

53

Extended Side Angle Pose (II)

Utthita Parsvakonasana

This more advanced variation of the Extended Side Angle Pose (see page 22) is deepened by moving the arms into new positions that extend the stretch while maintaining the stable and grounded "warrior" position of the legs, which should be familiar to you from the beginner's program.

The left arm is brought over the head to create a strong, unbroken, diagonal line along the side of the body. This lateral stretch strengthens the calves and thighs, corrects misalignments in the ankles and knees, trims the waist and hips, and expands the ribcage to facilitate deep breathing. The full extension of the posture also relieves back pain caused by arthritis or sciatica. However, you should not attempt it until you can comfortably sustain the less profound stretch of the beginner's posture.

54

DEEPENING THE STRETCH
Place one hand on the floor to deepen the lateral alignment of the body. Begin by aiming to place the hand on the outside of your foot, although as you progress you may be able to place it on the inside edge so that your upper arm pushes your knee outward.

Foundation Posture

Extended Side Angle Pose (I)

— TAKE CARE —

Practice the posture against a wall to learn correct alignment. Focus on remaining as two-dimensional as possible. As you look up, keep your neck lengthened and avoid tilting your chin up. Turn your chin toward your shoulder.

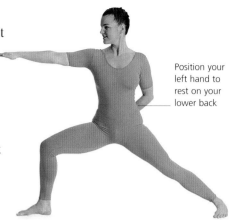

1 From Mountain Pose, step your feet 4¹/₂ft apart and extend your arms out to the sides. Your feet should be positioned so that they are directly beneath the palms of your hands.

Your heels should be aligned with each other and your toes should be facing forward

2 Bend your right knee so that your thigh and calf form a right angle with each other. Your right leg should be bent at the knee, with your thigh parallel to the floor, and your left leg should be straight and extended. Turn your head to look along your extended right arm and drop your left arm behind your back.

Position your left hand to rest on your lower back

3 Exhale and bring your right hand down to the floor, either inside or outside your front foot. Aim to place your palm flat on the floor but start with just your fingertips. Straighten your back leg and press your foot flat into the floor. As you inhale, pull back your left shoulder, open your chest, and look up at the ceiling. Imagine that you are practicing the pose against a wall and try to keep your body as two-dimensional as possible.

Do not drop your head

Keep your pelvis centered and facing forward

4 Exhale and stretch your left arm up and over your head so that it forms a diagonal line with your leg. Turn your left palm down and look under your left arm, up toward the ceiling. Keep your back foot pressed flat to the floor.

✳ *Hold for 10 breaths.*

▷ *Repeat the sequence on the other side and return to the Mountain Pose.*

Extended Foot Pose (II)

Prasarita Padottanasana

This posture is extended from the beginner's version (see page 24) into a cycle of movements made up of two modifications of the basic pose. As you progress in your practice, attempt to thread the postures together with your breath so that you move fluidly from one variation into the next.

By widening the legs and deepening the forward bend, this sequence of linked movements develops and tones the leg muscles and increases flexibility in the lower back and hips. In particular, the first variation adds a stretch through the arms that encourages greater flexibility in the shoulders and upper back. The increased degree of inversion also brings the benefits of mental and emotional calm. Always begin your practice of the extended variations by performing the basic *asana* once through and make sure that you have mastered the foundation posture before you move on to the more advanced variations.

DEEPENING THE STANCE
Prasarita is the Sanskrit word meaning "spread out" or "expanded" and it indicates the greater distance between the feet that intensifies the stretch from the beginner's variation.

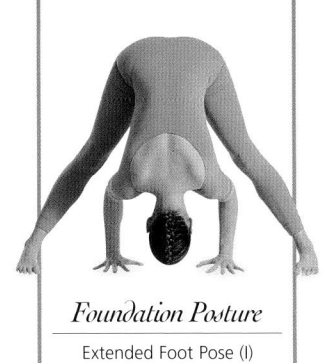

Foundation Posture
Extended Foot Pose (I)

— TAKE CARE —

Keep your legs straight and strong and your feet parallel to each other.

Relax and lengthen your neck during the posture, especially in the second variation.

Do not perform intensely inverted postures if you suffer from high blood pressure.

56

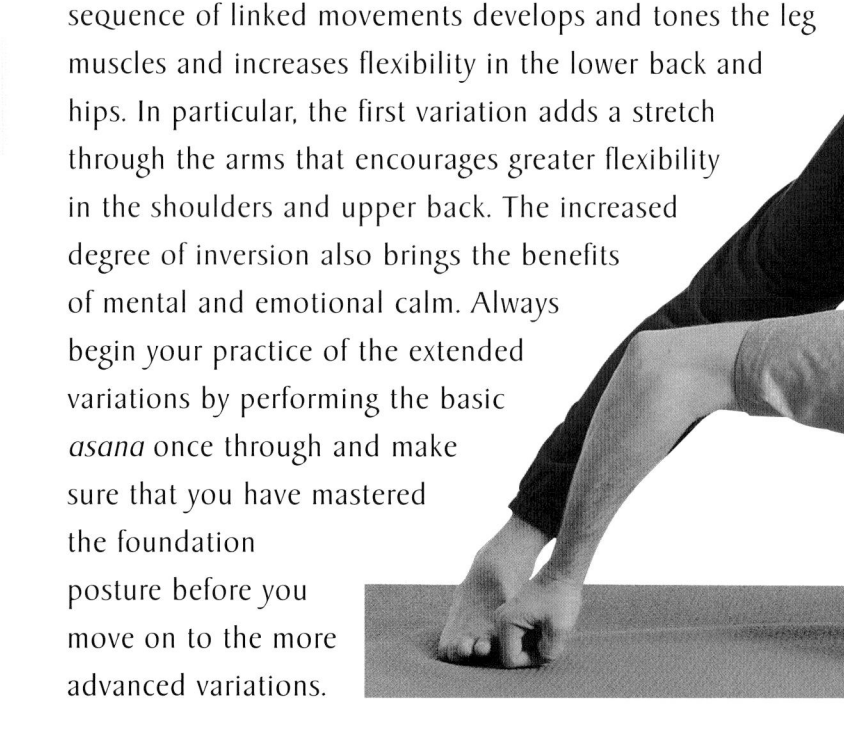

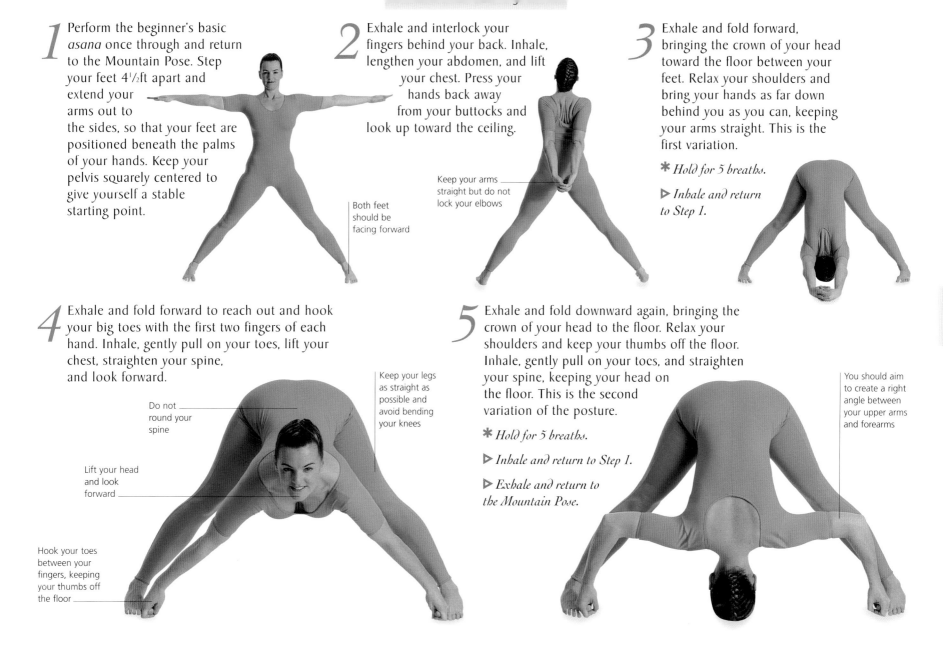

1 Perform the beginner's basic *asana* once through and return to the Mountain Pose. Step your feet 4¹/₂ft apart and extend your arms out to the sides, so that your feet are positioned beneath the palms of your hands. Keep your pelvis squarely centered to give yourself a stable starting point.

Both feet should be facing forward

2 Exhale and interlock your fingers behind your back. Inhale, lengthen your abdomen, and lift your chest. Press your hands back away from your buttocks and look up toward the ceiling.

Keep your arms straight but do not lock your elbows

3 Exhale and fold forward, bringing the crown of your head toward the floor between your feet. Relax your shoulders and bring your hands as far down behind you as you can, keeping your arms straight. This is the first variation.

✱ *Hold for 5 breaths.*

▶ *Inhale and return to Step 1.*

4 Exhale and fold forward to reach out and hook your big toes with the first two fingers of each hand. Inhale, gently pull on your toes, lift your chest, straighten your spine, and look forward.

Do not round your spine

Lift your head and look forward

Hook your toes between your fingers, keeping your thumbs off the floor

Keep your legs as straight as possible and avoid bending your knees

5 Exhale and fold downward again, bringing the crown of your head to the floor. Relax your shoulders and keep your thumbs off the floor. Inhale, gently pull on your tocs, and straighten your spine, keeping your head on the floor. This is the second variation of the posture.

✱ *Hold for 5 breaths.*

▶ *Inhale and return to Step 1.*

▶ *Exhale and return to the Mountain Pose.*

You should aim to create a right angle between your upper arms and forearms

57

Tree Pose (II)

This variation intensifies the beginner's posture (see page 26) by bringing the raised foot into the Half Lotus position. This opens the hip and knee joints but also requires greater flexibility than the basic posture. It also requires a high degree of concentration to perform properly, so take your time and do not rush into it. Always focus your mind before performing the posture by practicing *drushte* (steady gazing) at a fixed point for a few moments to achieve mental and physical calm. The Lotus Pose is an important posture for meditation (see page 92) and the Tree Pose with the foot in the Half Lotus position develops mental equilibrium as well as physical balance.

If you are supple and have mastered this posture, you may extend it further by introducing an intense forward bend over the supporting foot. The raised foot is held in Half Lotus by the right hand and the left hand is placed on the floor for stability. This posture is called *Ardha Baddha Padangushtasana*, the Half Bound Foot Big Toe Pose. It adds the mentally calming benefits of inversion and also massages the abdominal organs. This is a much more advanced posture and is included to indicate ways in which postures can be combined as you progress. However, you should not attempt it until you are well practiced and confident.

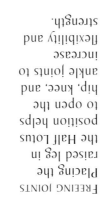

FREEING JOINTS
Placing the raised leg in the Half Lotus position helps to open the hip, knee, and ankle joints to increase flexibility and strength.

Foundation Posture
Tree Pose (I)

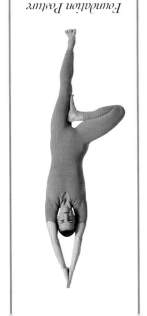

— TAKE CARE —

It is essential to work from the hip and not to force the knee.

If your legs and hips are very tight, gently swing your legs and shake out your feet to relax them before and after performing the posture.

If the posture places too much pressure on your knees, remain in the beginner's posture until you are ready to progress.

58

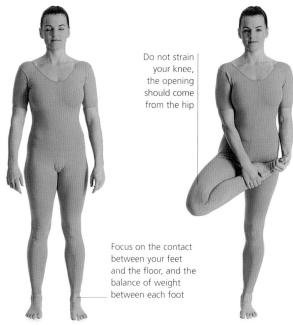

Do not strain your knee, the opening should come from the hip

Focus on the contact between your feet and the floor, and the balance of weight between each foot

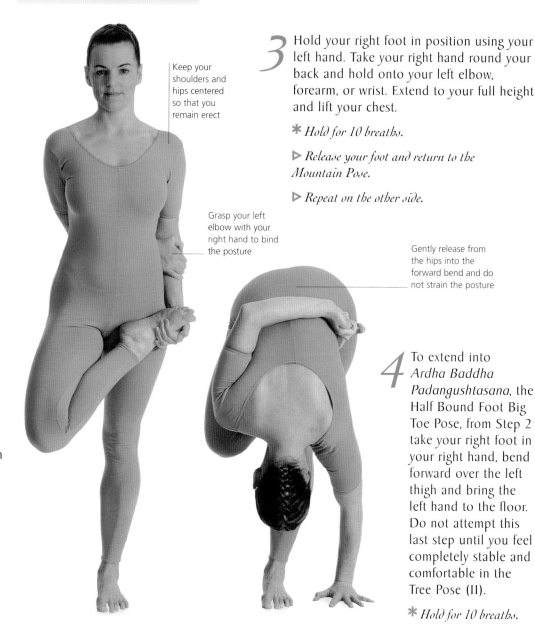

Keep your shoulders and hips centered so that you remain erect

Grasp your left elbow with your right hand to bind the posture

Gently release from the hips into the forward bend and do not strain the posture

1 Begin by stepping your feet approximately hip-width apart and relaxing your arms by your sides. Close your eyes and try to remain as steady as possible by focusing on the even distribution of weight between your feet. With practice, you should eventually be able to remain steady with your eyes closed in the Mountain Pose.

2 Open your eyes and gaze at a point about 15ft ahead of you for a few moments. Raise your right foot and grasp it, placing it as high up as possible on your left thigh. Inhale and gently lift your right heel toward your navel. Exhale, and as you do so, carefully lower your right knee toward the floor.

3 Hold your right foot in position using your left hand. Take your right hand round your back and hold onto your left elbow, forearm, or wrist. Extend to your full height and lift your chest.

✱ *Hold for 10 breaths.*

▷ *Release your foot and return to the Mountain Pose.*

▷ *Repeat on the other side.*

4 To extend into *Ardha Baddha Padangushtasana*, the Half Bound Foot Big Toe Pose, from Step 2 take your right foot in your right hand, bend forward over the left thigh and bring the left hand to the floor. Do not attempt this last step until you feel completely stable and comfortable in the Tree Pose (II).

✱ *Hold for 10 breaths.*

59

Hurdler's Pose

Triang Mukhaikapada Paschimottanasana

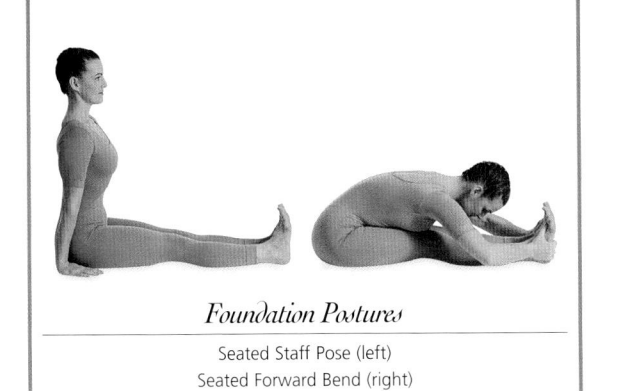

Foundation Postures

Seated Staff Pose (left)
Seated Forward Bend (right)

This is the first of the more advanced seated forward bends that are demonstrated in the intermediate program. Before you attempt it, you should always perform the basic foundation postures (see pages 28–31). *Triang* means "three parts" or "limbs" and refers to the foot, knee, and buttock of the folded leg. *Mukhaikapada* means "facing one foot" and refers to the forward bend over the extended leg. The Hurdler's Pose opens the hips and knees, tones the abdominal organs, and increases the circulation of blood to the pelvis to keep the reproductive organs healthy. By pressing the top of the foot into the floor and positioning the heel toward the ceiling, the Hurdler's Pose also helps to correct fallen arches, relieves ankle sprains, and realigns the knees and hips.

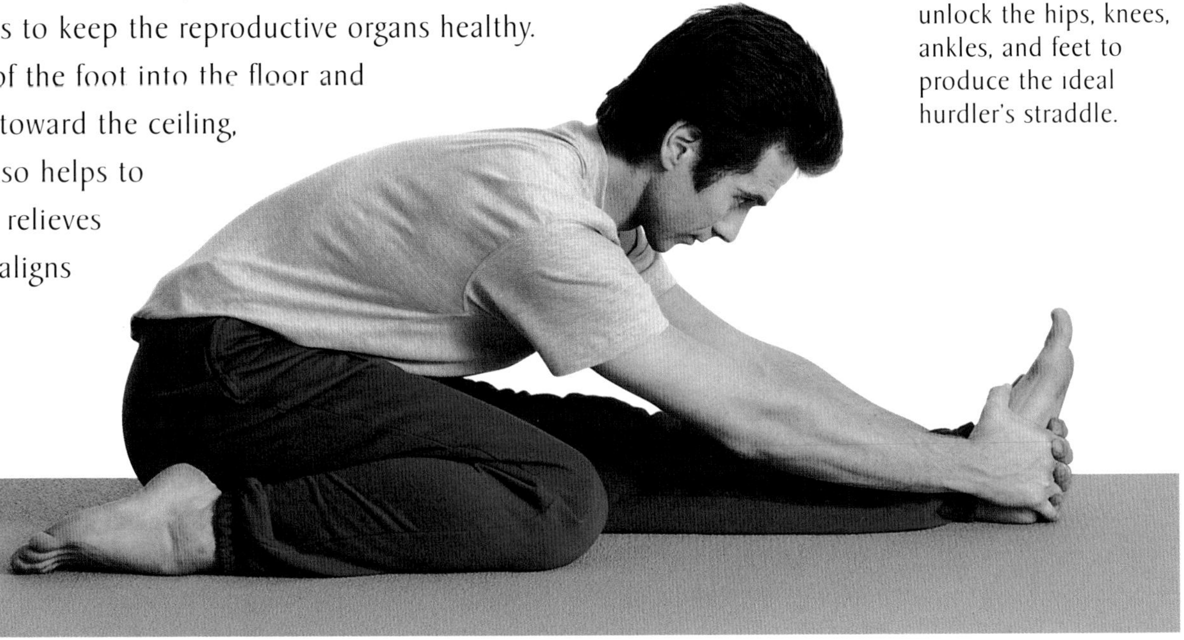

OPENING THE JOINTS
This posture may seem intense at first but perseverance will unlock the hips, knees, ankles, and feet to produce the ideal hurdler's straddle.

TAKE CARE

If you find that you fall excessively to your left, place your left hand on the floor by your side and fold forward with your right hand only.

Always realign your body by performing the Staff Pose and the basic Seated Forward Bend before practicing any of the more complex variations.

▼ *If you find that your hips or knees are particularly stiff, place a 2-inch thick yoga block or large book under your left buttock to perform the posture.*

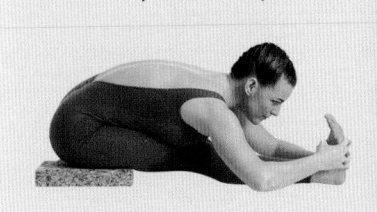

60

1 From the Staff Pose, fold your right leg back so that the top of your right foot is resting on the floor on the outside edge of your right buttock. Position the folded leg so that, if possible, both buttocks are on the floor and the knees are drawn together.

2 Adjust your posture by taking the thumb of your right hand behind your knee and rolling your calf muscle out to the side. Lift your left buttock out to the side to ensure you are positioned correctly on your sitting bones. Inhale, reach up toward the ceiling, and look at your thumbs.

3 Exhale, reach forward, and grasp your left ankle or heel with both hands if possible. Inhale, pull on your left heel, lift your torso, and straighten your arms.

Look forward as you lengthen your torso

Flex your toes toward the ceiling

4 Exhale, fold forward, and bring your chin toward your left knee. Keep your spine straight and your shoulders level. Try to bring your right buttock down to the floor without straining your knee.

✳ *Hold for 10 breaths.*

▷ *Return to Step 3.*

▷ *Exhale, release, and repeat on the other side.*

61

Keep your thighs parallel with each other

Relax your shoulders away from your ears and focus on releasing tension in your shoulder blades

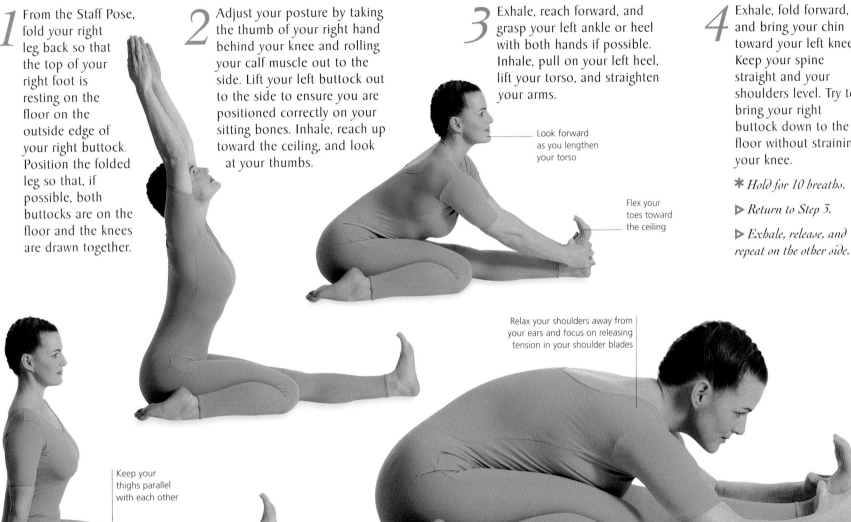
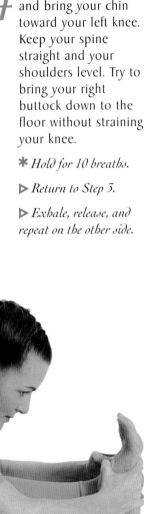

Half Lotus Seated Forward Bend

Ardha Baddha Padma Paschimottanasana

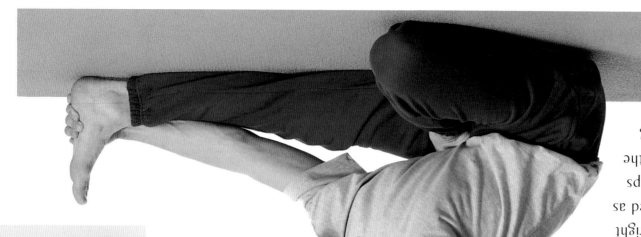

If your hips are flexible, you may find this variation, which places the legs alternately in Half Lotus, a comfortable position in which to work. For others, it may require more practice and you should not force your body into the posture. Placing the feet in the Half Lotus position encourages a deep opening of the hip, knee, and ankle joints, and with regular practice you may become flexible enough to sit comfortably in the classic yoga posture of the Lotus Pose.

In the full posture, the right arm is brought behind your back to take hold of the right foot. This binds the posture and is used as a lever to deepen the bend. It also helps to open the shoulder joint, as well as the hip. Binding the full posture by linking your limbs increases your awareness of your physical posture and improves the coordination between different systems of your body.

CIRCULATION AND DIGESTION
Pressing the heel lightly into the abdomen gives the internal organs a gentle massage.

— TAKE CARE —

Always realign your body in the Staff Pose and practice the basic Seated Forward Bend before trying a harder variation. In Half Lotus, make sure you place your foot high up into the hip with the heel pointing toward your navel, and do not force your knee.

▲ *If the intermediate posture strains your joints, practice the beginner's One Leg Seated Forward Bend, but intensify it by grasping the heel with your hand.*

1 Perform the Staff Pose to realign the body. From here, place your right foot as high up on your left thigh as is comfortably possible, without straining your knee. Inhale, reach up, and look up toward your thumbs.

Keep your arms straight but do not lock your elbows

Keep your spine straight and do not slump

2 Exhale, fold forward, and grasp your left ankle or heel with both hands. Try to stretch through to your fingertips as you reach forward. As you inhale, pull on your heel, straighten your arms, extend your torso, and look up.

Bring your right shoulder down so that it is level with your left shoulder

Grip the toe of your right foot between your fore and index fingers

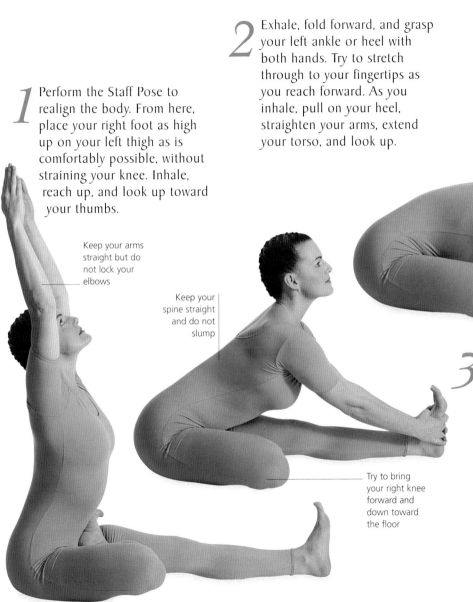
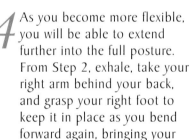

Try to bring your right knee forward and down toward the floor

3 Exhale and fold forward, keeping your spine straight, and bring your chin toward your left knee. Keep your chest lifted and open and your shoulders away from your ears. Try to bring your right shoulder level with your left shoulder.

* *Hold for 10 breaths.*

▷ *Inhale and return to Step 2.*

▷ *Return to the Staff Pose and repeat on the other side.*

4 As you become more flexible, you will be able to extend further into the full posture. From Step 2, exhale, take your right arm behind your back, and grasp your right foot to keep it in place as you bend forward again, bringing your chin toward your knee.

* *Hold for 10 breaths.*

▷ *Inhale and return to Step 2.*

▷ *Return to the Staff Pose and repeat on the other side.*

63

Seated Spinal Twist (II)

This posture, which is named after the yogic sage *Marici*, is a progression from the beginner's twisting posture *Matsyendrasana*, the Seated Spinal Twist (I) (see page 36). *Marichyasana*, the Seated Spinal Twist (II), increases the degree of movement put through the spine to encourage maximum flexibility in the back and to increase stimulation of the central nervous system.

The twisting movement has a number of benefits for the digestive system as it provides a healthy massage for the intestines and abdominal organs. It also strengthens the neck, opens the shoulders, and releases tension in the hips. This makes it a particularly good posture to practice if much of your day is spent in a sedentary position. The binding in the full extension of the posture acts as a lever to deepen the twist further. However, you should not attempt it until you have gained sufficient spinal mobility through practice of the basic posture.

64

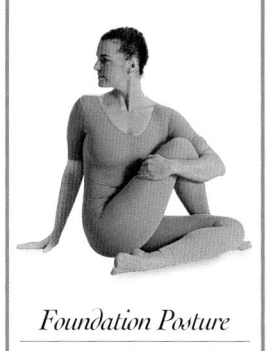

Foundation Posture

Seated Spinal Twist (I)

STEADY PROGRESS
Do not rush to achieve the full posture but work steadily and deeply, with sensitivity to your body's capabilities and needs.

—— TAKE CARE ——

As you twist, always lengthen your spine, lift up and out of your sitting bones, lift your chest, and open your shoulders.

Keep your neck long and lift your ears away from your shoulders.

Keep the foot of your straight leg flexed toward the ceiling.

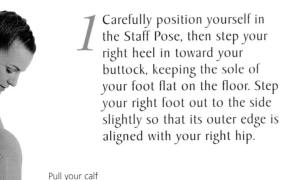

1 Carefully position yourself in the Staff Pose, then step your right heel in toward your buttock, keeping the sole of your foot flat on the floor. Step your right foot out to the side slightly so that its outer edge is aligned with your right hip.

Pull your calf into your body as far as possible

Keep your foot flexed toward the ceiling

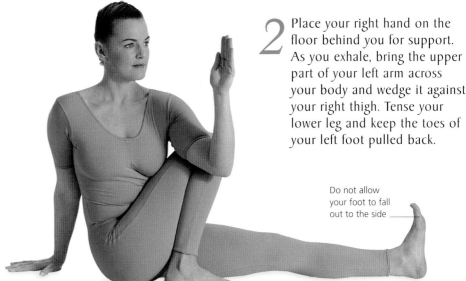

2 Place your right hand on the floor behind you for support. As you exhale, bring the upper part of your left arm across your body and wedge it against your right thigh. Tense your lower leg and keep the toes of your left foot pulled back.

Do not allow your foot to fall out to the side

65

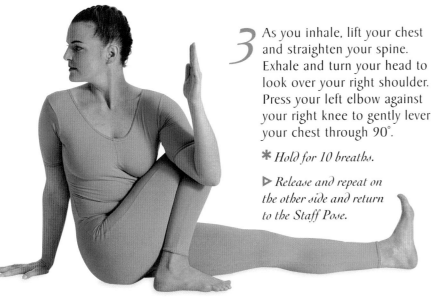

3 As you inhale, lift your chest and straighten your spine. Exhale and turn your head to look over your right shoulder. Press your left elbow against your right knee to gently lever your chest through 90°.

* *Hold for 10 breaths.*

▷ *Release and repeat on the other side and return to the Staff Pose.*

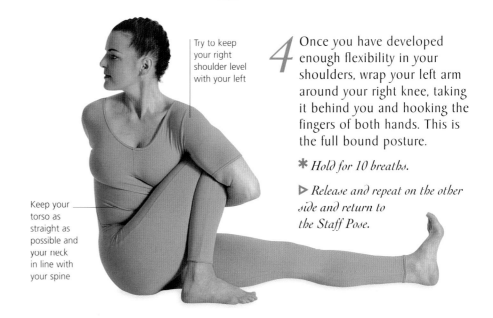

Try to keep your right shoulder level with your left

Keep your torso as straight as possible and your neck in line with your spine

4 Once you have developed enough flexibility in your shoulders, wrap your left arm around your right knee, taking it behind you and hooking the fingers of both hands. This is the full bound posture.

* *Hold for 10 breaths.*

▷ *Release and repeat on the other side and return to the Staff Pose.*

Butterfly Pose

Baddha Konasana

The literal translation of the Sanskrit name *Baddha Konasana* is the Bound Angle Pose. However, the posture is more commonly known as the Butterfly Pose because the angle of the legs—bent at the knees, with the thighs pressed close to the floor, bound and tucked as far as possible into the pelvis—resembles a butterfly's open wings.

The Butterfly Pose has a stretching effect on the inner thighs and hips and encourages the flow of blood to the pelvis, abdomen, and back. It helps counteract the effects of a sedentary lifestyle by maintaining the health of the spine, kidneys, and (in men) the prostate gland. It is also a beneficial posture for women because it helps maintain a healthy menstrual cycle, guards against problems affecting the urinary tract, and is useful during pregnancy, easing lower-back pain and opening the hips to prepare the body for giving birth.

COBBLER'S POSE
The deep opening of the hips in this posture counters the problems of sitting for many hours at a time. For this reason, shoemakers in India practice their craft in this position, giving the posture its second alternative name.

TAKE CARE

Maintain a straight spine as you lean forward to avoid straining your upper back. Keep the front of your chest lifted and your shoulders open as you bend from the hips.

Be aware of your breathing as you practice the posture, making sure you inhale and exhale evenly and deeply.

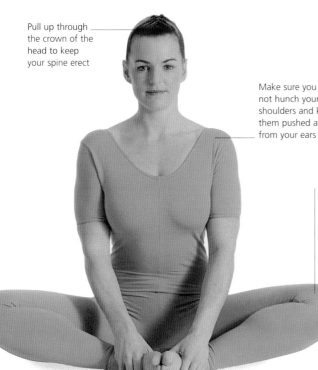

Pull up through the crown of the head to keep your spine erect

Make sure you do not hunch your shoulders and keep them pushed away from your ears

Through regular practice you will eventually be able to bring your knees all the way to the floor

To prevent slumping in this posture, look forward and do not drop your head

Try not to hunch your shoulders

Eventually you may be able to bring your chin to the floor

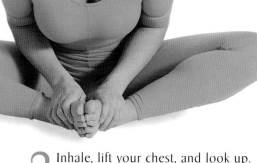

Push your legs together to take out the stretch

1 From the Staff Pose bring the soles of your feet together, dropping your knees out to the sides. Grip your feet and gently pull your heels in toward your groin without forcing them. Inhale, lift your chest, straighten your spine, and drop your chin slightly. Continue to pull gently on your feet and press your knees toward the floor.

❋ *Hold softly for 10 breaths.*

2 Inhale, lift your chest, and look up. Exhale and fold forward from your lower back. Take your chin forward and down toward your feet as far as is comfortable. Look up and extend your torso forward.

❋ *Hold for 10 breaths.*

3 To counterpose the posture, inhale, come back up, squeeze your knees together, and relax for a few moments before continuing your practice.

Wide Leg Seated Forward Bend

Literally translated from the Sanskrit, *Upavistha Konasana* means "seated angle pose." This indicates the deep opening of the hip and sacrum in this posture, which stimulates the circulation of blood to the pelvis. Like the Butterfly Pose (see page 66), it helps keep the female reproductive system healthy and can be particularly beneficial for women who suffer from painful periods.

Once you are familiar with the posture and aware of your level of flexibility, you may wish to practice a variation of this pose with another person. Your partner must also practice yoga and you should make sure that both of you are conscious of each other's physical limits. Face your partner and spread your legs apart, keeping your feet flexed and touching each other's. Join hands and slowly roll in a circular movement, first one way and then the other, as if stirring a great mixing bowl. Be attentive to your partner's movements and abilities and concentrate on your breathing as you practice the posture in order to achieve a fluid and graceful motion or *vinyasa*. Do not force your body into the full extension of the posture as it takes time to develop the requisite flexibility. Regular and gentle practice will reap the most beneficial and safest results.

Hamstring health
In this posture, the legs are kept straight and the feet flexed, both of which give a deep stretch to your hamstrings and your lower back.

68

— TAKE CARE —

Do not force or strain as you practice in this posture. Breathe deeply, keep your spine as straight as possible, and lift out of your sitting bones as you bend.

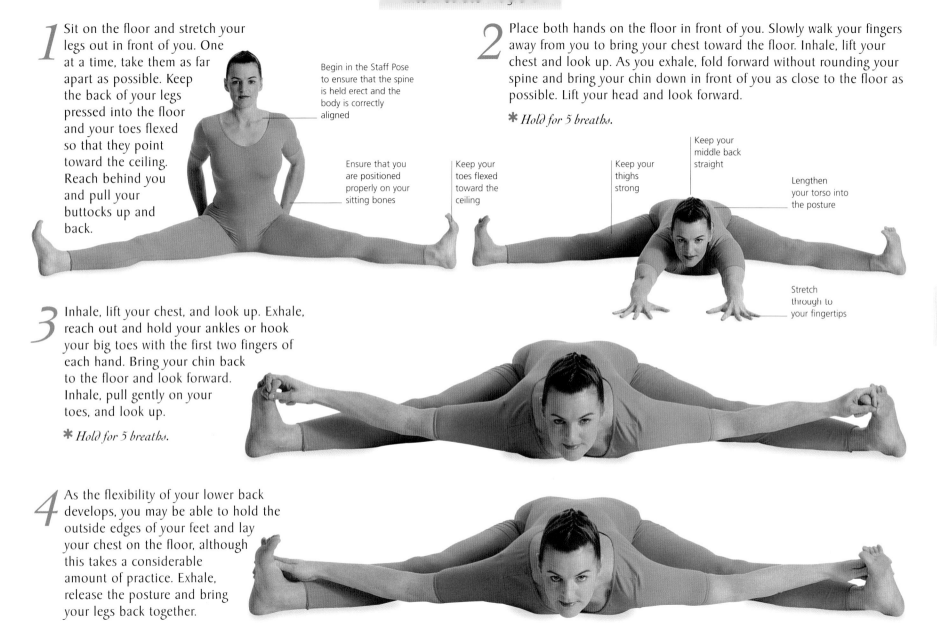

1 Sit on the floor and stretch your legs out in front of you. One at a time, take them as far apart as possible. Keep the back of your legs pressed into the floor and your toes flexed so that they point toward the ceiling. Reach behind you and pull your buttocks up and back.

Begin in the Staff Pose to ensure that the spine is held erect and the body is correctly aligned

Ensure that you are positioned properly on your sitting bones

Keep your toes flexed toward the ceiling

2 Place both hands on the floor in front of you. Slowly walk your fingers away from you to bring your chest toward the floor. Inhale, lift your chest and look up. As you exhale, fold forward without rounding your spine and bring your chin down in front of you as close to the floor as possible. Lift your head and look forward.

✱ *Hold for 5 breaths.*

Keep your middle back straight

Keep your thighs strong

Lengthen your torso into the posture

Stretch through to your fingertips

3 Inhale, lift your chest, and look up. Exhale, reach out and hold your ankles or hook your big toes with the first two fingers of each hand. Bring your chin back to the floor and look forward. Inhale, pull gently on your toes, and look up.

✱ *Hold for 5 breaths.*

4 As the flexibility of your lower back develops, you may be able to hold the outside edges of your feet and lay your chest on the floor, although this takes a considerable amount of practice. Exhale, release the posture and bring your legs back together.

69

Upward Dog Pose

Urdhva Mukha Svanasana

This posture resembles a dog stretching up onto its front legs and extending its hind legs behind it, hence its name, which translates as "upward" (*urdhva*), "facing" (*mukha*), "dog pose" (*svanasana*). It may be seen as a companion posture to the Downward Dog Pose (see page 40), as it encourages a deep back bend in the spine and stretches the entire front of the body from the chin to the feet. It is also part of the Sun Salutation sequence (see page 50).

The Upward Dog Pose is an extension of the Cobra Pose (see page 38). The basic *asana* is intensified by coming onto the toes to deeply arch and lift the whole body from the floor, supported only by the hands and the tops of the feet. Upward Dog thus develops both upper body strength and flexibility, relieves backache, and opens the chest and throat to encourage deep breathing.

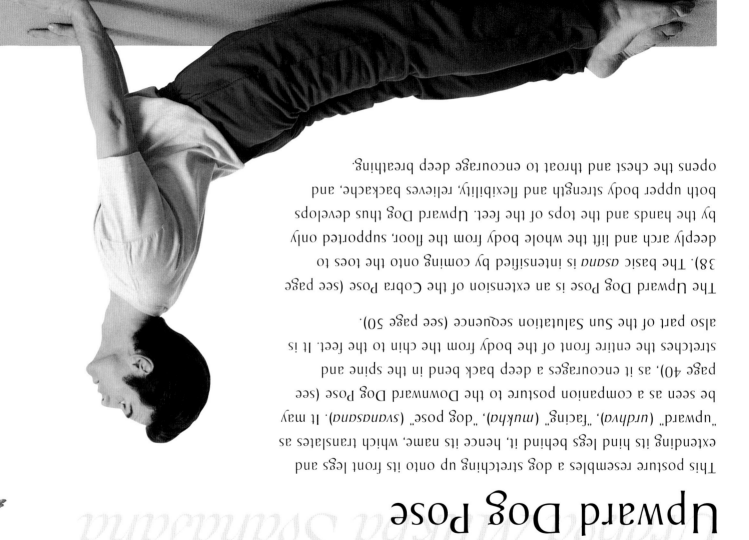

FLUID MOVEMENT

This posture forms part of the dynamic Sun Salutation warm up, and regular practice will help you perform the entire sequence more smoothly and with greater control.

Foundation Posture
Cobra Pose

TAKE CARE

Stretch from the tips of your toes through your legs to your spine to avoid straining the lower back.

Avoid hunching your shoulders and aim to maintain a graceful curve of the spine by keeping the arms stable and straight.

Counterpose either in the Child Pose or by lying on your stomach to release the spine.

1 Start on your hands and knees with your elbows directly beneath your shoulders. Keep your fingers spread out and your middle fingers facing forward.

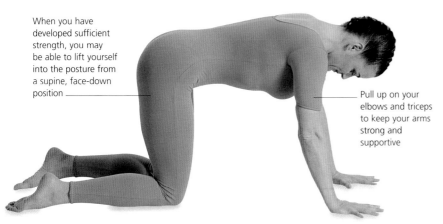

When you have developed sufficient strength, you may be able to lift yourself into the posture from a supine, face-down position

Pull up on your elbows and triceps to keep your arms strong and supportive

2 Keep your hands in place and your arms firm. Step your feet out behind you, one at a time, into *Caturanga Dandasana*, or the Sloping Plank Pose, which also makes up part of the Sun Salutation. Keep your feet hip-width apart and your toes tucked under.

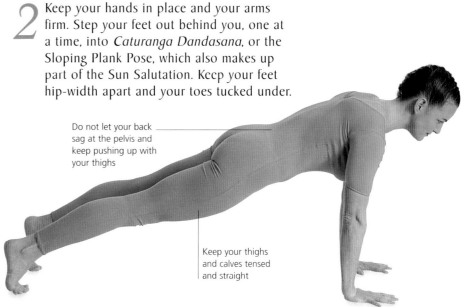

Do not let your back sag at the pelvis and keep pushing up with your thighs

Keep your thighs and calves tensed and straight

3 Inhale, roll over your toes, bend your back, and open your chest. Try to keep your knees and thighs off the floor and imagine your back making a smooth curve from the base of your spine to your skull. To extend the stretch, turn your head and look back at your heels.

✻ *Hold for 3 breaths.*

Lift your chin and look toward the ceiling but ensure that you do not close down the back of your throat

Focus on releasing the tension in your shoulder blades to avoid hunching your shoulders and to maximize the stretch in your spine

4 Exhale, release the posture, and lie down flat on your stomach. Place both hands under your head and rest the side of your face in your hands.

✻ *Rest for 5 breaths.*

▷ *Return to Step 1.*

▷ *Repeat the whole sequence twice more.*

Alternate which side of your face you lay in your hands as you repeat the sequence

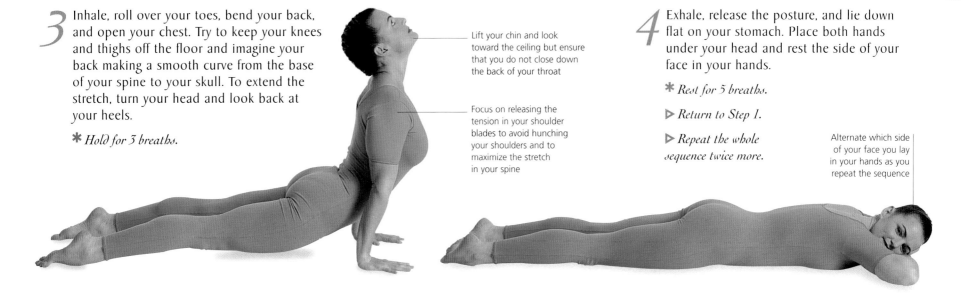

Locust Pose

Salabhasana

In this posture, the body is made to resemble a locust that has alighted on the ground. Hence the name *Salabhasana*, meaning Locust Pose. It provides a wonderful stretch for the back, making it an ideal counterposture to any of the forward bends in this program. The posture encourages elasticity in the spine and is particularly beneficial for people suffering from slipped discs or general back pain.

There are many internal benefits of the Locust Pose: the expansion of the chest can be extremely helpful to people with asthma or other respiratory problems, while balancing on the front of the abdomen aids digestion, relieves trapped wind, and encourages the efficient function of the bladder and, in men, the prostate gland. At first, you may find that you are unable to lift your legs very far off the floor. Regular, steady practice will gradually increase the degree of lift of which you are capable.

TAKE CARE

▼ *If you suffer from lower back pain, keep your toes together but move your thighs apart slightly and bend your knees. This will relieve pressure in your lower back.*

Do not practice the Locust Pose if pregnant.

TAKE YOUR TIME
The Locust Pose is a much more intense stretch than it appears to be. Follow the steps carefully and slowly to avoid straining your back.

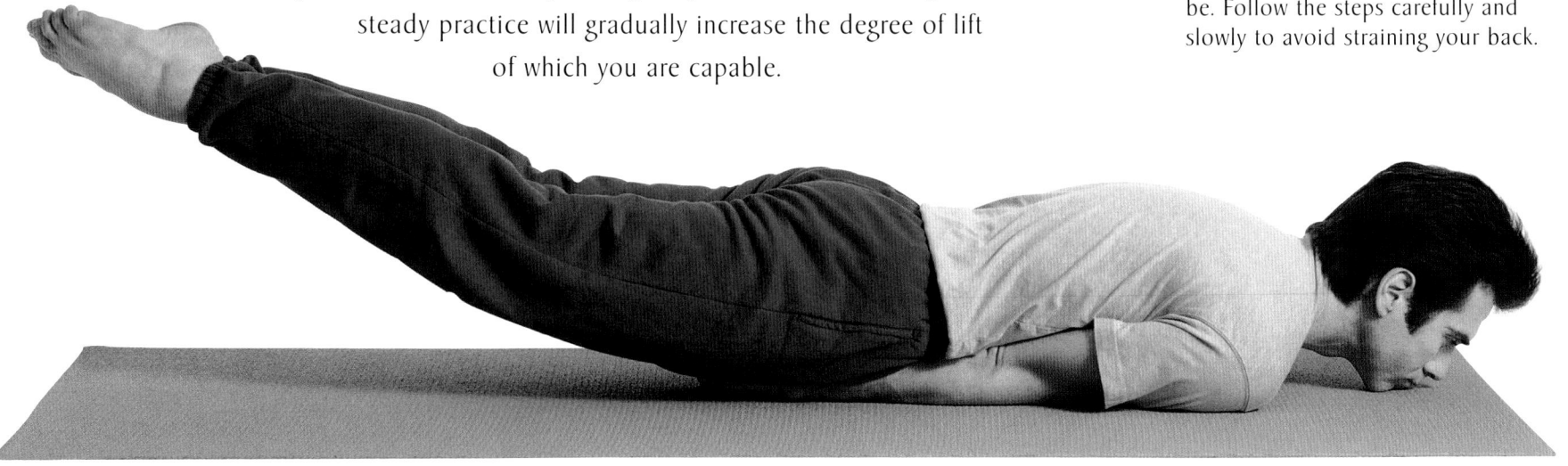

72

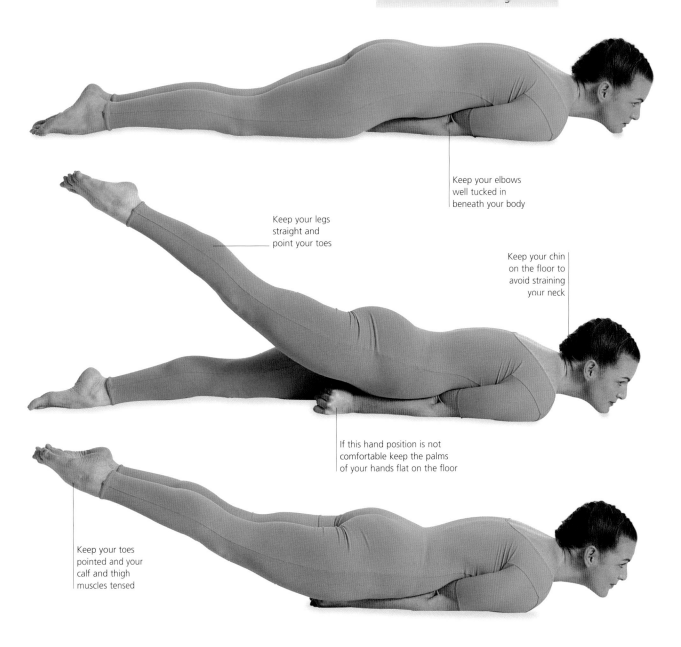

Keep your elbows well tucked in beneath your body

Keep your legs straight and point your toes

Keep your chin on the floor to avoid straining your neck

If this hand position is not comfortable keep the palms of your hands flat on the floor

Keep your toes pointed and your calf and thigh muscles tensed

1 From the Child Pose move to lie on your front. Roll onto your side and make fists with your hands, then bring them together in front of you. Roll back onto your front with your arms tucked beneath you, work your elbows together under your body, and rest your chin lightly on the floor.

2 Inhale, press into the floor with your hands, and lift your right leg as high as you can. Point your toes and try not to swivel or tilt your hips.

   ✶ *Hold for 5 breaths.*

   ▷ *Release and repeat on opposite leg.*

   ▷ *Rest briefly and repeat once again on both sides.*

3 Work your elbows a little closer together under your body and lift both legs at the same time. The degree of lift of which you are capable will increase greatly with practice.

   ✶ *Hold for 5 deep breaths.*

   ▷ *Exhale and return to the Child Pose.*

   ✶ *Rest for 10 breaths.*

Bow Pose
Dhanurasana

This posture is so-called because the arms are used to create a bow-string that lifts the torso and legs simultaneously, producing a deep, backward curve of the spine.

This posture strengthens the muscles of your back and stretches the entire length of the front of your body, from your chin to your toes. Your shoulders are pulled back to open the front of your chest and thus improve lung capacity. Ideally, the knees and feet should be kept together, but this takes a lot of practice. Instead, concentrate on pushing the abdomen into the floor, while lifting the buttocks. Try to enter into and release the posture smoothly and avoid making any abrupt or jerky movements that might aggravate the spine. Perform this posture after intense spinal stretches or twists, as the back bend in the Bow Pose is supported by both the arms and the abdomen.

CORRECT TECHNIQUE
Feel the stretch all the way along your spine. Try to keep your arms light and relaxed, not rigid.

74

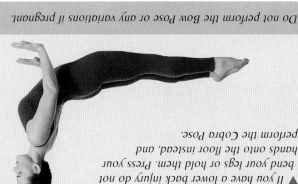

— TAKE CARE —

▲ If you have a lower back injury do not bend your legs or hold them. Press your hands onto the floor instead, and perform the Cobra Pose.

Do not perform the Bow Pose or any variations if pregnant.

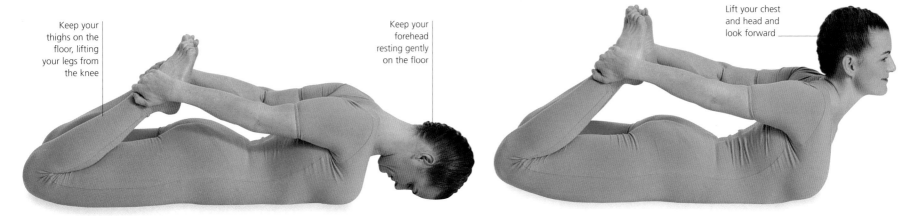

Keep your thighs on the floor, lifting your legs from the knee

Keep your forehead resting gently on the floor

Lift your chest and head and look forward

75

Pull your shoulders back to open the chest

Keep your arms straight but do not lock the elbows

Do not allow your knees to fall further than hip-width apart

1 Lie down on your stomach and rest your forehead on the floor. Reach back and grasp your ankles, or if you can't reach them, hold your feet, keeping your toes touching.

2 Slowly and gently pull against your feet, lifting your chest and head as you do so. Look straight ahead and keep your arms straight in the posture.

3 Inhale, push your feet away from you, and allow your knees and thighs to rise off the floor.

＊ *Hold this posture for 5 breaths.*

▷ *Exhale and return to Step 1.*

▷ *Rest briefly and repeat Steps 2 and 3 twice.*

＊ *Rest in the Child Pose for 10 breaths.*

Headstand

Sirsasana

This reviving inversion brings about a feeling of lightness and exhilaration, as healthy, oxygen-rich blood flows to the brain. This powerful posture has many positive remedial effects and it is often called "the king of all *asanas*" because of its numerous and diverse mental, emotional, and physical benefits.

Sirsasana, the Headstand, nourishes the brain and in particular the pituitary and pineal glands that are responsible for energy levels and vitality. Many people believe that regular practice can sharpen intellectual ability, increase memory, and enhance powers of concentration. The inversion of this posture also provides physical benefits: it cleanses the internal organs by returning blood to the heart, soothes the digestive tract to ease bowel disorders, strengthens the respiratory system, and invigorates the circulation. It is also a beneficial posture to practice if you suffer from varicose veins. The Headstand is an intense posture and can take some time to master fully. You may find it helpful to gradually work up to the full posture by concentrating on achieving each individual stage first, rather than tackling the sequence as a whole. Perseverance with this challenging *asana* is rewarded with a heightened sense of both physical balance and psychological equilibrium.

BUILDING ABILITY

The most intense of the inverted postures shown in this book, you should only attempt the Headstand once you feel comfortable maintaining the Half Shoulderstand.

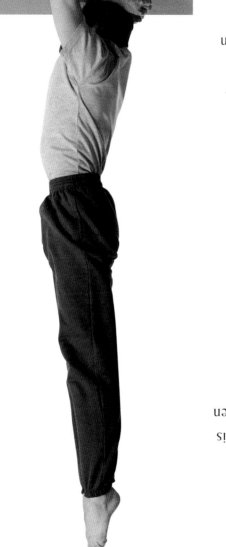

▲ *Always practice against a wall at first. From the Child Pose, walk your feet slowly up the surface. As you gain confidence, use the wall only as a safety net until you are ready to try it unaided.*

TAKE CARE

Set your arm position carefully before beginning and keep the majority of your weight distributed from your elbows to your wrists, with only minimal pressure placed on your head and neck.

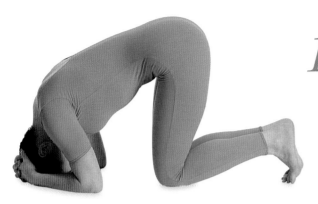

1 Kneel down and place your forearms and elbows in front of you (wrap your fingers loosely around your elbows to find the correct distance apart). Keeping your elbows in position, place your hands on the floor. Interlock your fingers, keeping your palms open. Place the crown of your head on the floor and push the back of your head firmly into your open palms.

4 When you have mastered the second stage, raise your bent knees up toward the ceiling and allow your feet to drop back behind you. This is stage three.

2 Lift your knees off the floor and come up onto your toes, taking as much weight as you can on your forearms. Walk your feet toward your face and allow your hips to move backward to keep your neck in line with your spine. Transfer your weight so that you can lift your legs approximately 2 inches from the floor.

3 When you have mastered the first stage, slowly bring your knees a little closer into your chest and raise your heels toward your buttocks. This is the second stage.

5 Finally, bring your feet all the way up toward the ceiling into the full posture. Never come out of the Headstand hurriedly, but release the posture gradually, coming through the same stages in reverse to avoid dizziness.

✳ *Hold for 30 breaths.*

▷ *Rest in the Child Pose for 15 breaths.*

77

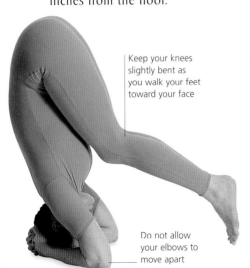

Keep your knees slightly bent as you walk your feet toward your face

Do not allow your elbows to move apart

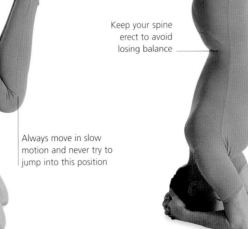

Always move in slow motion and never try to jump into this position

Keep your spine erect to avoid losing balance

Relax your face, keep your shoulders away from your ears, and breathe deeply

Shoulderstand to Plough Pose

Sarvangasana to Halasana

Like the Headstand (see page 76), *Sarvangasana* or the Shoulderstand has a wide range of rejuvenating effects: it revives the internal organs, soothes the brain, enhances concentration, and provides a deep inversion that is a tonic for the entire system. The Shoulderstand is often seen as the companion posture to the Headstand and is consequently known as the "Queen of all *asanas*." From the Shoulderstand, you move smoothly into the Plough Pose by dropping your legs behind your head. This encourages flexibility in the spine, releases tension in the shoulders, improves circulation, and massages the abdomen.

You should not attempt this sequence until you have mastered the beginner's Half Shoulderstand (see page 44).

HEALING INVERSIONS
As with the other inverted postures, the Plough Pose increases blood flow to the brain to enhance mental clarity and equilibrium.

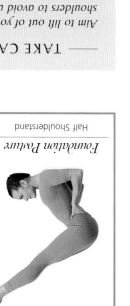

Foundation Posture
Half Shoulderstand

TAKE CARE

Aim to lift out of your shoulders to avoid unnecessary stress being placed on the neck. Never turn your head while in this posture.

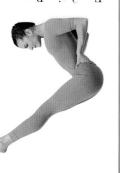

▲ If you cannot touch your toes to the floor in the Plough Pose, curl up your legs and firmly support your back with your hands.

Do not practice the Shoulderstand if you suffer from high blood pressure.

78

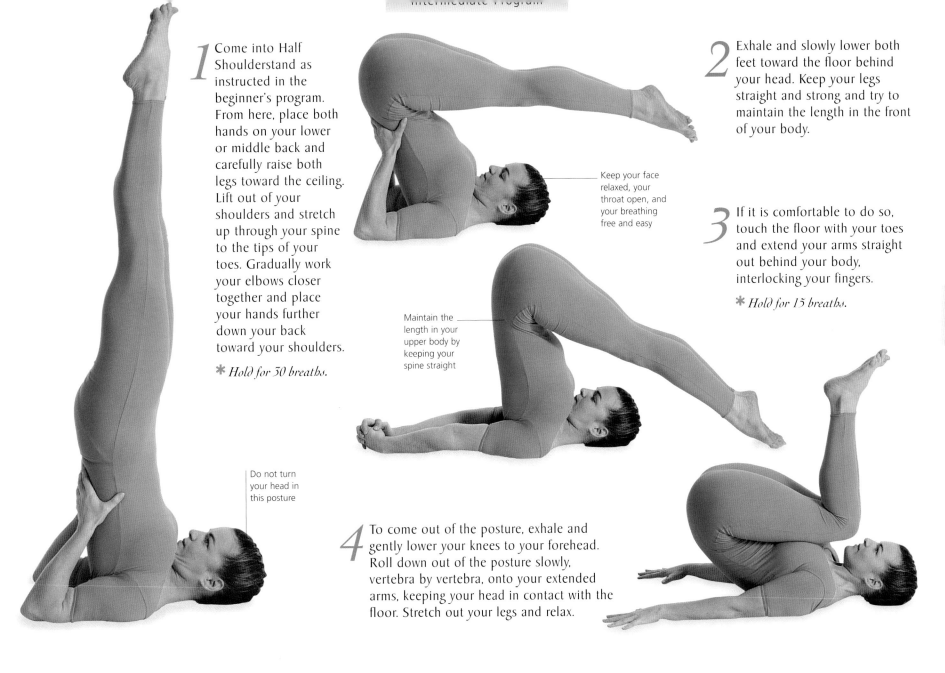

1 Come into Half Shoulderstand as instructed in the beginner's program. From here, place both hands on your lower or middle back and carefully raise both legs toward the ceiling. Lift out of your shoulders and stretch up through your spine to the tips of your toes. Gradually work your elbows closer together and place your hands further down your back toward your shoulders.

✻ *Hold for 30 breaths.*

Do not turn your head in this posture

Keep your face relaxed, your throat open, and your breathing free and easy

2 Exhale and slowly lower both feet toward the floor behind your head. Keep your legs straight and strong and try to maintain the length in the front of your body.

3 If it is comfortable to do so, touch the floor with your toes and extend your arms straight out behind your body, interlocking your fingers.

✻ *Hold for 15 breaths.*

Maintain the length in your upper body by keeping your spine straight

4 To come out of the posture, exhale and gently lower your knees to your forehead. Roll down out of the posture slowly, vertebra by vertebra, onto your extended arms, keeping your head in contact with the floor. Stretch out your legs and relax.

Fish Pose (II)

Matsyasana

This extended variation of the basic Fish Pose (see page 46) is a wonderful counterposture to the intense spinal stretches and contractions of the Shoulderstand to Plough Pose sequence (see page 78).

The opening of the chest provided by the beginner's posture is broadened in this variation by folding the arms and bringing them behind the head, so that the elbows rest on the floor. This stretches the intercostal muscles (which are situated between the ribs) and expands the capacity of the ribcage and lungs. The efficiency of the respiratory system is thus increased, making it a great posture for athletes.

The Fish Pose (II) requires flexibility and may take some time to master. Once you have built sufficient strength, you may wish to extend the posture further into the advanced Outstretched Foot Pose, which develops from the Fish Pose by lifting the arms and legs off the floor.

STEADY PROGRESS
You have to be flexible in order to place your elbows on the floor in this posture. Ease yourself into the extension gradually and at your own pace.

Foundation Posture

Fish Pose (I)

TAKE CARE

If you have a stiff neck or neck problems, perform the beginner's posture or modification.

Try to lift your chest as high off the ground as you can to expand your ribcage and encourage deep breathing.

When you drop your head back, keep your head and face completely relaxed.

80

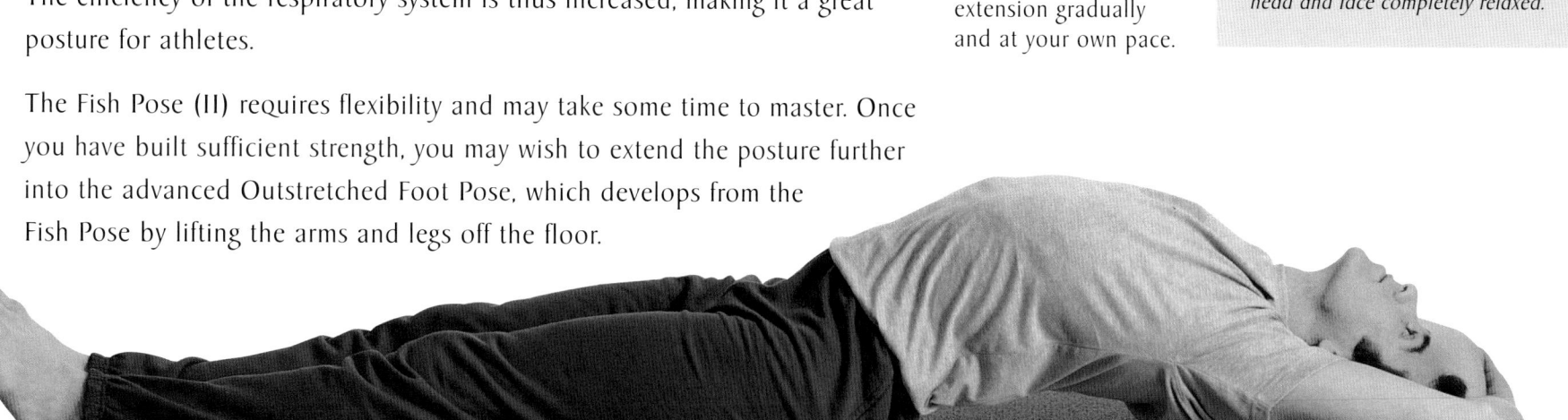

1 Beginning in the Corpse Pose, lift up onto your forearms and transfer your weight onto your elbows. Keep your head upright, with your chin toward your chest. You should be familiar with this preparatory position from the beginner's program.

Keep your elbows close together

Keep your feet and legs together and do not allow your feet to fall outward

2 Tuck your head under and bring the crown of your head to rest gently on the floor. Breathe deeply into the top of your chest. This is the full extent of the beginner's posture.

* *Hold for a few moments.*

Gaze toward the middle of your forehead

3 From the basic posture, stretch out your arms behind your head and clasp your elbows in your hands. Relax your elbows gently toward the floor as you do so. This is the full posture.

* *Hold for 15 breaths.*

* *Counterpose by bringing your chin to your chest and resting for 5 breaths.*

▶ *Return to the Corpse Pose.*

Continue to breathe deeply into the clavicular top chest

81

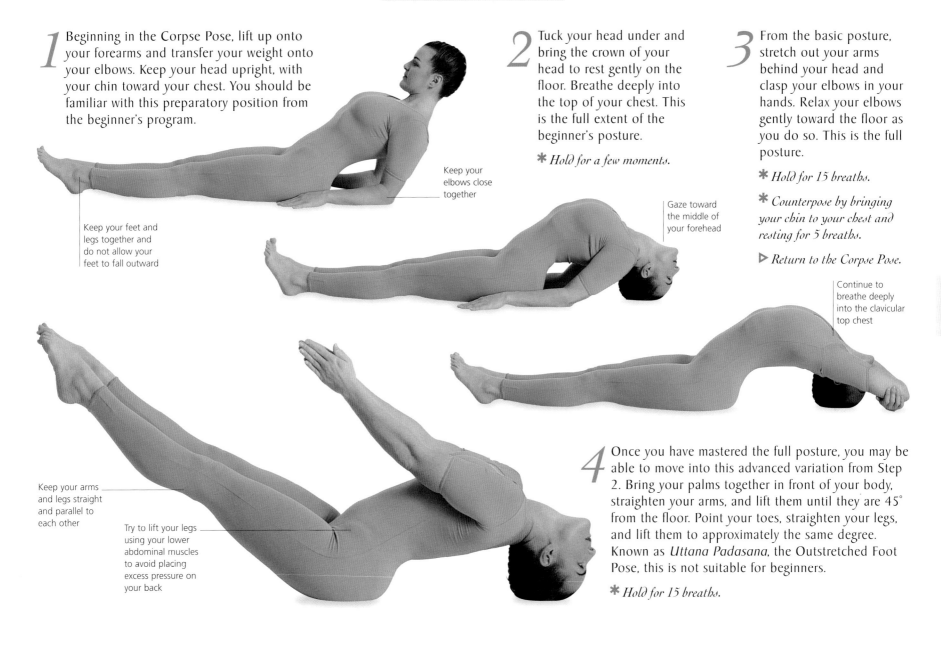

Keep your arms and legs straight and parallel to each other

Try to lift your legs using your lower abdominal muscles to avoid placing excess pressure on your back

4 Once you have mastered the full posture, you may be able to move into this advanced variation from Step 2. Bring your palms together in front of your body, straighten your arms, and lift them until they are 45° from the floor. Point your toes, straighten your legs, and lift them to approximately the same degree. Known as *Uttana Padasana*, the Outstretched Foot Pose, this is not suitable for beginners.

* *Hold for 15 breaths.*

Yoga Breathing Exercises

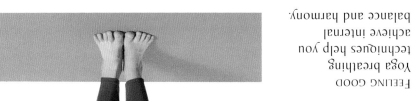

Breathing properly is essential not only for your physical well-being; it also helps to calm the mind and channel the flow of vital energy through the body. Learning to control your breath is therefore an integral part of yogic practice.

BREATHING YOURSELF FIT *Prana* is Sanskrit for both breath and life; it is the universal energy that flows through all living things. *Ayama* means expansion, stretching, or restraint. *Pranayama* is therefore the extension and control not only of the breath, but of vitality, and even of life itself. Yogic breathing brings balance to the emotions, clarity to the mind, and rejuvenation to the body.

Mastery of some *pranayama* techniques is more difficult than others and incorrect or unsupervised practice of the more complex yoga breathing exercises could be harmful. However, certain simple techniques can be practiced by the novice as well as the more experienced yoga student, provided you begin gradually. Some techniques appear deceptively easy, so if you become faint or dizzy you should stop immediately and breathe normally. You can practice the breathing exercises shown on the following pages immediately before your yoga session to help clear your mind and energize your body in preparation for

physical exertion. However, they can be equally effective outside your yoga workout—to help you relax if you feel stressed.

When performing *pranayama*, your lungs should be fully expanded. To do this, you must sit in a position that keeps your spine erect and your chest open, such as the Easy Pose, the Half Lotus or, if you can maintain it comfortably, the full Lotus Pose. These postures are symmetrical and grounded, and therefore encourage both physical and mental balance.

FEELING GOOD Yoga breathing techniques help you achieve internal balance and harmony.

82

Pumping Breath

Kapalabhati literally means "shining skull;" practicing this technique makes your eyes shine and your face glow, clears your mind, and enhances your powers of concentration. As well as being a *pranayama*, *kapalabhati* is also considered to be a *kriya* or cleansing practice for the lungs. During this dynamic breathing exercise, the stale air that usually lingers in the lower lobes of the lungs is forcibly exhaled and fresh, oxygen-rich air is allowed to enter the body, contributing to the rejuvenating and invigorating effects of the technique. As your lung capacity gradually increases, you will eventually be able to work up to sixty pumping breaths per round. Regular practice of *kapalabhati* not only increases lung capacity but also tones your stomach muscles and is beneficial for the cardiovascular system and the liver. If you feel faint or become short of breath at any time, stop and breathe normally.

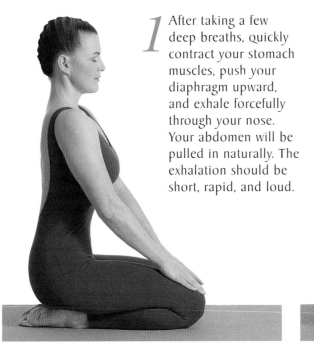

1 After taking a few deep breaths, quickly contract your stomach muscles, push your diaphragm upward, and exhale forcefully through your nose. Your abdomen will be pulled in naturally. The exhalation should be short, rapid, and loud.

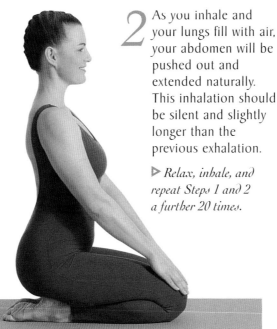

2 As you inhale and your lungs fill with air, your abdomen will be pushed out and extended naturally. This inhalation should be silent and slightly longer than the previous exhalation.

▷ *Relax, inhale, and repeat Steps 1 and 2 a further 20 times.*

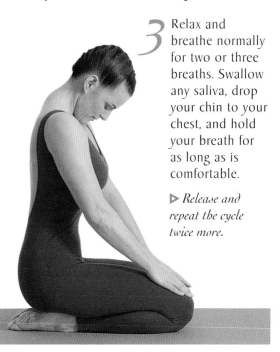

3 Relax and breathe normally for two or three breaths. Swallow any saliva, drop your chin to your chest, and hold your breath for as long as is comfortable.

▷ *Release and repeat the cycle twice more.*

83

Victorious Breath

Ujjayi Pranayama translates from the Sanskrit as Victorious Breath and refers to the way in which the chest swells, to resemble a warrior, on each inhalation when performing this exercise.

The first principle of the Victorious Breath is to inhale and exhale through your nose and channel the air directly into your lungs. Concentrate on the rise and fall of your chest and the lateral expansion of your ribcage out to the sides and into your back as you inhale. The second principle is that the exhalations are as active as the inhalations. Keep your in- and out-breaths the same length and try to maintain a continuous rhythm without pausing when your lungs are fully inflated or deflated. The third principle is to narrow the back of your throat so that as your breath passes over your larynx and vocal chords it produces a hissing sound. This ensures that your full lung capacity is utilized and more energy-giving oxygen is absorbed into your bloodstream.

You can energize your yoga sessions by using this technique throughout your posture practice. It is especially useful during dynamic, *vinyasa* sequences of movements. Begin by standing in the Mountain Pose and take a few Ujjayi breaths to awaken your system before you embark on your routine of postures.

84

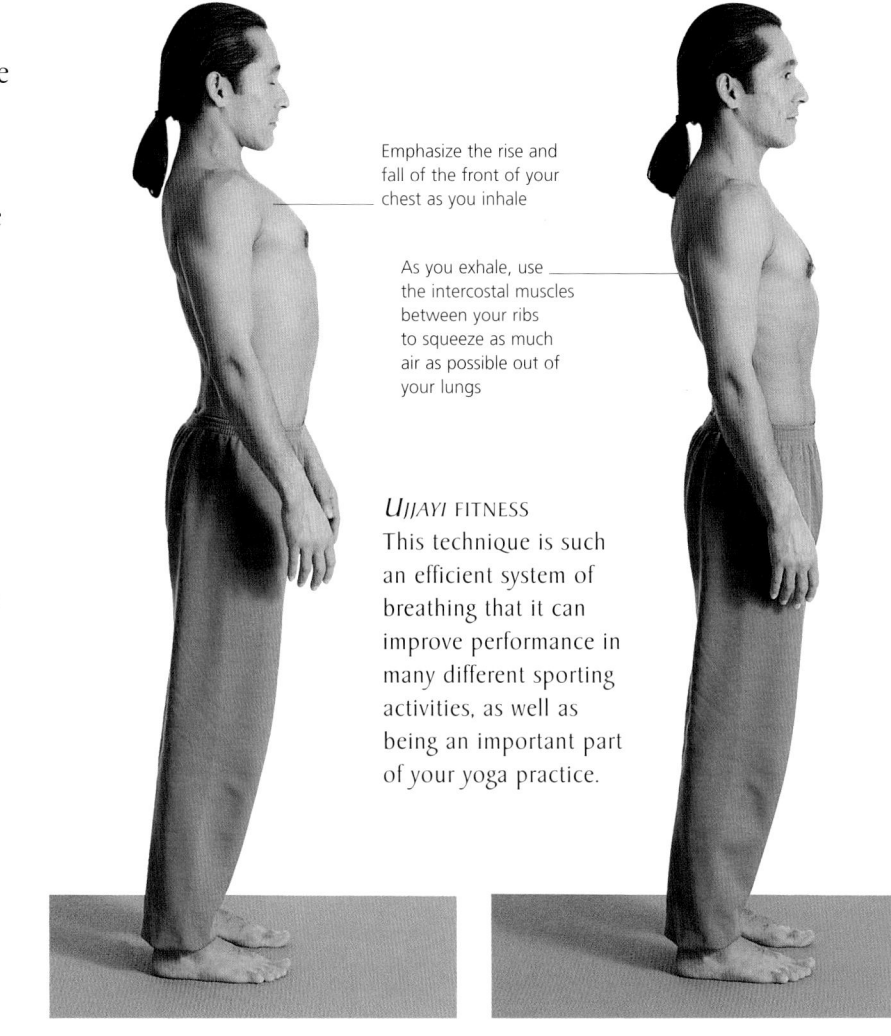

Emphasize the rise and fall of the front of your chest as you inhale

As you exhale, use the intercostal muscles between your ribs to squeeze as much air as possible out of your lungs

UJJAYI FITNESS
This technique is such an efficient system of breathing that it can improve performance in many different sporting activities, as well as being an important part of your yoga practice.

Alternate Nostril Breathing

Anuloma Viloma

This is a more advanced *pranayama* and requires some practice to master. However, it is extremely beneficial for the respiratory system and helps balance the flow of energy in the body. *Anuloma* means "with the natural order," while *viloma* means "going against" it. This refers to the way in which the technique channels the breath through alternate nostrils, so that energy is made to flow equally through the *ida* and *pingala nadi* (see pages 88–9). What's more, it unites the left and right hemispheres of the brain, encouraging increased efficiency in the function of every system in the body. The respiratory system also benefits because the exhalations are twice as long as the inhalations, so that stale air and toxins are expelled from the lungs.

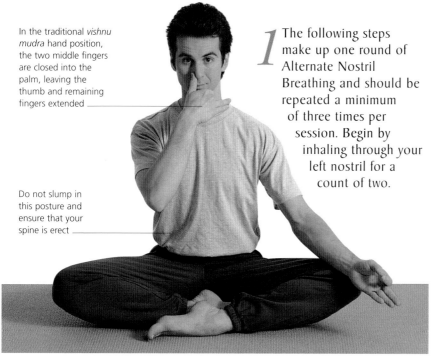

In the traditional *vishnu mudra* hand position, the two middle fingers are closed into the palm, leaving the thumb and remaining fingers extended

Do not slump in this posture and ensure that your spine is erect

1 The following steps make up one round of Alternate Nostril Breathing and should be repeated a minimum of three times per session. Begin by inhaling through your left nostril for a count of two.

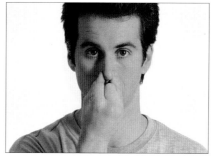

2 Keeping your right nostril closed with your thumb, seal your left nostril using your little and ring fingers. Hold this position and retain your breath for a count of eight.

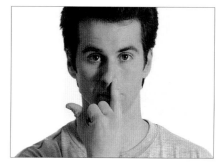

3 Take your thumb away and exhale through your right nostril for a count of four. Inhale through the same nostril and again close both nostrils and hold your breath for a count of eight. Exhale through your left nostril.

▶ *Return to Step 1.*

THE YOGA WAY OF LIFE

Yoga is not simply a system of exercise: it can be a whole way of life. According to the philosophy behind yoga, the poses are but one of eight disciplines. To reap the full benefits of yoga, you may like to practice it in the context of these other seven aspects.

The postures demonstrated in this book are only a preparatory stage in the wider-reaching system of hatha yoga. Practicing the *asanas* brings many benefits, purifying the body and maintaining its health. But to experience the full scope of yoga's benefits, the postures should be practiced together with the other aspects of hatha yoga, such as meditation, concentration, and healthy eating, some of which are introduced over the following pages.

YOGA PHILOSOPHY As a combination of science, physical discipline, and practical philosophy, yoga is considered a complete system for living. It originated in India thousands of years ago, but despite its antiquity it is just as relevant in the modern world.

Of the many practitioners to have written treatises systematizing the different strands of yoga over the millennia, the legendary yogi Patanjali is the best known. Thought to have lived some time between 400 BC and AD 400, this ancient Himalayan philosopher and yogi was an authority on medicine and grammar, as well as yoga. Patanjali is credited with devising the principles or *sutras* that mark the path or *sadhana* toward spirituality in yoga. The threads of his wisdom have survived by word of mouth through generations to form the basis of the contemporary practice of hatha yoga.

THE SYMBOLIC TREE Patanjali's authoritative and influential text is called the *Yoga Sutras*. Available today, it sets out a program for attaining physical and spiritual fulfillment. According to this treatise, yoga consists of eight equally important branches or limbs that graduate in a symbolic tree.

The limbs of this tree are interrelated but each is worked through sequentially to reach the ultimate goal of yoga—*samadhi*, a creative and transcendent state where the mind is completely still. Translated from Sanskrit as "absorption," *samadhi* refers to the enlightened state of supreme consciousness and union.

THE EIGHT LIMBS OF YOGA According to Patanjali's teachings, each branch or limb of the tree must be attempted and conquered by students of yoga in order for them to achieve their full physical and spiritual potential, and thereby attain lasting peace.

The first two limbs of Patanjali's tree are a collection of moral laws or ethics by which a yogi should live his life. The *yamas* or abstentions form the first branch and consist of five moral injunctions. They promote the principles of honesty, non-violence, control of bodily desire, non-possessiveness, and non-stealing. The second limb, known as the *niyamas* or observances, are the ethical laws that govern the behavior of the yoga student. These include rules of austerity, purity, contentment, selflessness, and dedication.

The following two limbs are the practice of yoga postures *(asanas)* and breathing exercises *(pranayama)*. The intensity of the yoga poses teaches mastery of the body through physical discipline, while the breathing exercises encourage a strong respiratory system and teach the student of yoga to harness the living force or *prana* within us all. You have encountered some of the techniques of yogic breathing on pages 82–5. Mastery of the first four limbs leads the yoga student to the higher limbs, which focus on the internal being.

THE WHEEL OF LIFE
The wheel is a traditional Eastern metaphor for the eternal cycle of life. The eight spokes correspond to the eight limbs of Patanjali's tree in hatha yoga, leading to eternal enlightenment or *samadhi*.

The fifth limb, withdrawal from the material world *(pratyahara)*, distances the yogi from external distractions. This is followed by concentration *(dharana)*, which disciplines the mind so that it becomes single-pointed and properly focused. This opens the door to meditation *(dhayana)*, the seventh limb, which allows the yogi to achieve a state of profound mental and emotional calm and to focus on the inner person or soul. The meditative state is believed to enable the yogi to look beyond *maya*, the illusory power of the physical world, in order to perceive and comprehend a greater truth. The final branch of Patanjali's tree is the achievement of union with the universal, which is also translated as enlightenment. The last three limbs, *dharana*, *dhayana*, and *samadhi*, are together called *samyama*, the internal limbs.

THE PATH TO ENLIGHTENMENT According to Patanjali, only when each of these eight limbs have been sequentially conquered can the yogi achieve enlightenment, and therefore reach his full potential as a human being. An introduction to yogic physiology and the way energy travels through our bodies, some concentration and meditation exercises, and advice on how to fuel your body according to yogic principles are explored in detail on the following pages to help you extend your yoga practice.

The Subtle Body

Pranayama Kosha

According to yoga philosophy, the physical body is merely the vehicle for an inner existence or soul. More important is the "subtle" body, or *pranayama kosha*, which surrounds the physical body through its many energy channels and centers. The practice of yoga is believed to activate the functions of the subtle body.

Just as the lower limbs of Patanjali's tree are focused on the physical body, the higher limbs are focused on the subtle body. The anatomy of the subtle body consists of the seven energy centers or *chakras*, and more than 70,000 energy channels or *nadis*. By learning to control your breathing, and through the physical discipline of the yoga postures, you can master the energies coursing through your body and eventually fulfill your spiritual potential.

THE SEVEN CHAKRAS Translated from Sanskrit as "wheels" or "circles," *chakras* are energy centers that connect the subtle body to the physical body. They store all the energy or life force (*prana*), the release of which is controlled through the breath (see pages 82–5). Each *chakra* is associated with a certain physical or emotional function and is also often associated with an element. All the *chakras* excepting the crown *chakra*, have their own mantras (see pages 92–3).

88

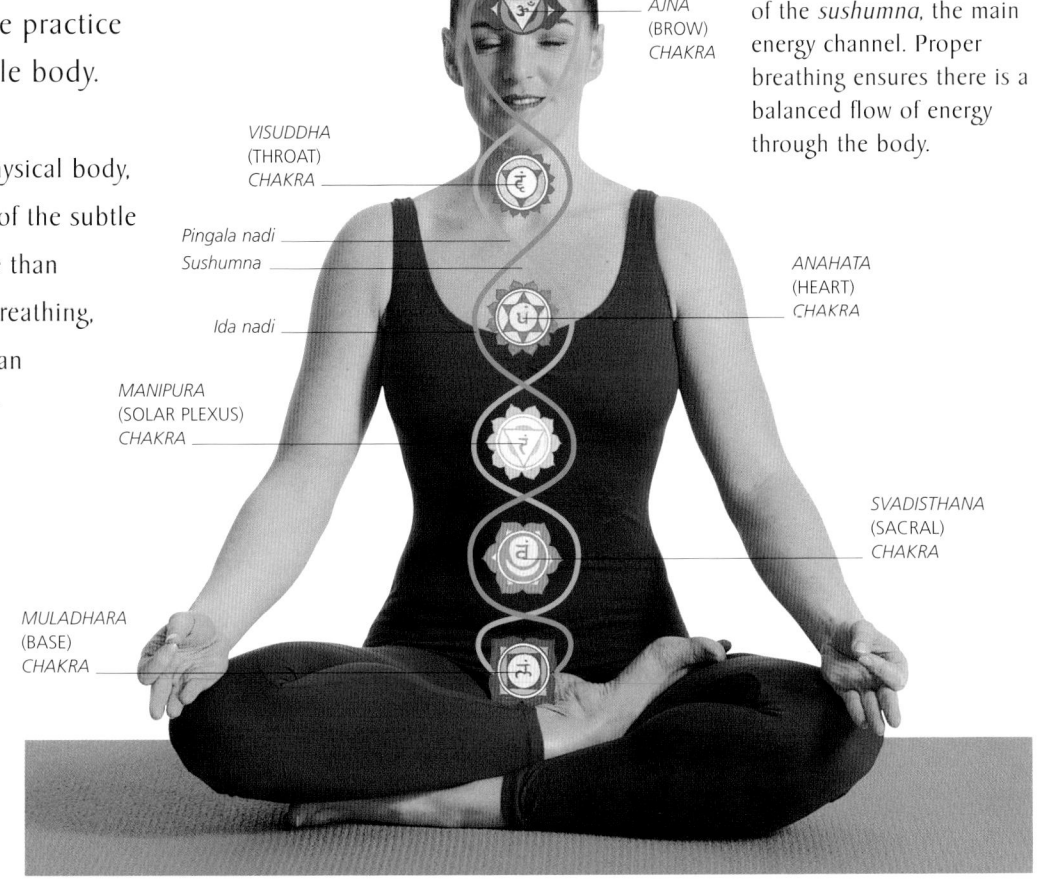

SAHASRARA (CROWN) CHAKRA

AJNA (BROW) CHAKRA

VISUDDHA (THROAT) CHAKRA

Pingala nadi

Sushumna

Ida nadi

MANIPURA (SOLAR PLEXUS) CHAKRA

ANAHATA (HEART) CHAKRA

SVADISTHANA (SACRAL) CHAKRA

MULADHARA (BASE) CHAKRA

AWAKENING THE BODY'S ENERGY
The seven *chakras* are positioned along the line of the *sushumna*, the main energy channel. Proper breathing ensures there is a balanced flow of energy through the body.

The seven major *chakras* are located at sequential intervals along the *sushumna*, the chief *nadi* or energy line that forms a vertical path along the spine. The first *chakra*, situated at the base of the spine, is the base or *muladhara chakra*. It means root or vital source and is associated with survival and the earth element. The sacral or *svadisthana chakra* (meaning "the abode of the soul") is the seat of sexuality and pleasure; its element is water. Next is the solar plexus or *manipura chakra*. Translated as "sun," this *chakra* is associated with fire, and controls the individual's will power, mental stamina, and emotional fortitude. The heart or *anahata chakra* means "unbeaten." It is associated with the triumph of love and compassion, and the air element. The throat or *visuddha chakra* governs intelligence and the creative spirit. The brow or *ajna chakra* is situated at the center of the forehead and is associated with perception and awareness. Last along the *sushumna* energy channel is the crown or *sahasrara chakra* (see illustration, right), which symbolizes eternity and opens to achieve wisdom and spiritual union.

MAPPING THE ENERGY CHANNELS The *nadis* form a network of energy channels throughout the subtle body. The primary *nadi* is the *sushumna*, which runs in a vertical column extending along the spine, connecting the seven *chakras*. Spiraling around either side of the *sushumna* are two secondary channels, the *ida nadi*

CROWN CHAKRA
All *chakras* are depicted as lotus flowers, with each petal symbolizing a certain physical or spiritual attribute. The crown *chakra* has a thousand petals, more than any of the other seven *chakras*, and represents wisdom and union.

(running from the left side of the base of the spine to the right nostril) and the *pingala nadi* (which runs from the right side of the base of the spine to the left nostril). The *ida* and *pingala nadis* govern opposing energies in the subtle body—sometimes described in terms of the polarity between male and female or yin and yang—similar to the way the left and right hemispheres of the brain control different functions in the physical body.

MAINTAINING THE BALANCE OF ENERGY According to most Eastern philosophies, an imbalance in these masculine and feminine energies can affect your physical and emotional well-being. Yoga postures and breathing techniques, such as Alternate Nostril Breathing (see page 85), can help to stimulate the activity of both the *ida* and *pingala nadis* to ensure an equal and balanced flow of energy around each side of the body. *Chakras* can be either open or closed. When yoga postures and breath are practiced, the life force or *prana* travels through the subtle body and stimulates successive *chakras* to open and release their energy. Each *chakra*'s energy is absorbed, right up until the crown *chakra* where the energy merges with a supreme state of consciousness and the yoga student reaches a state of spiritual enlightenment. Although you may be unaware of these esoteric energy systems, this energy flow will unconsciously be put into motion with consistent and steady practice of yoga *asanas* and *pranayamas*.

Concentration

Dharana

In order to achieve the ultimate goal of yoga—enlightenment—we must become immune to the distractions caused by our physical senses. To completely disengage the mind from its material preoccupations, however, requires highly developed powers of concentration.

The practice of *asanas* and *pranayamas* teaches physical discipline. This helps to temper the desires of the body that can otherwise prevent an individual from attaining emotional tranquility. Physical postures and breathing techniques must both be mastered before the yoga student may progress onto the higher limbs of Patanjali's tree (see page 87). These limbs consist of *pratyahara* or withdrawal, *dharana* or concentration, and *dhayana* or meditation.

The ancient Hindu text of the *Upanishads* describes the mind like a chariot pulled by a team of wild horses that need to be harnessed and controlled. The clamoring of our physical desires can pull our chariot off-course and only through physical and mental discipline can it be returned to the path. Concentration keeps the mind on course toward the ideal, positive state of *samadhi*. Because the mind wanders easily, you may like to try a traditional concentration technique such as focusing on your breathing or gazing at a visual stimulus (a technique known as *tratak*), as described on page 91.

OBSERVATION OF THE BREATH One of the simplest concentration techniques, this involves spending two or three minutes focusing on the physical sensations and rhythm of your breathing as it becomes slower and deeper. The increased oxygen intake relaxes your body, calms your thoughts, and heightens your awareness of the connection between body and mind.

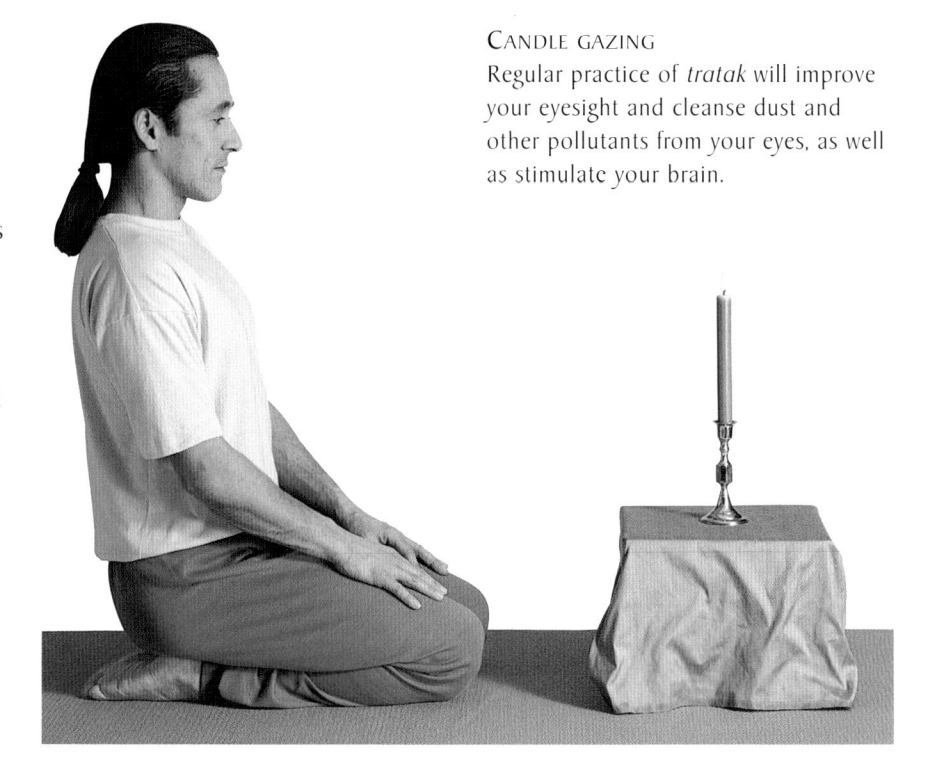

CANDLE GAZING
Regular practice of *tratak* will improve your eyesight and cleanse dust and other pollutants from your eyes, as well as stimulate your brain.

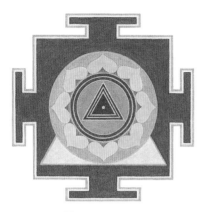

USING A YANTRA
Tratak can be performed using a visually striking object or image, such as a *yantra*, which means "tool" in Sanskrit. These traditional geometric symbols give abstract concepts a concrete form. Thus as the individual concentrates on the *yantra*, their mind is trained and focused on the image and the concept that it represents.

The aim of this exercise is to zero in on the sensations in your nose, mouth, lungs, and abdomen as you breathe steadily in and out. Don't try to force a rhythm on your breathing, just observe its natural pace and pauses. Counting your inhalations and exhalations in groups of five or ten will also keep you focused on your breathing and help prevent you from becoming distracted.

FOCUSING ON A VISUAL AID Another yoga concentration exercise is to gaze steadily at a visual stimulus in order to train the mind to a single concentrated point. This technique is known as *tratak*, and is traditionally performed by gazing at a candle flame. The light makes a strong impression on the eye and the image can be easily retained by the mind when the eyes are closed. It requires discipline to maintain a steady and focused gaze without allowing the eye and the mind to wander, however, and combined with the effort of retaining the mental image when the eyes are closed, *tratak* is an effective way of improving your powers of concentration. It may also be performed using a meaningful and visually striking image such as a *yantra* (see illustration above). The traditional detailed and colorful patterns of

these symbols make a similar impact on the eye as a candle flame and may be a more interesting or challenging image to retain mentally when your eyes are closed.

HOW TO PRACTICE TRATAK Place a lighted candle about 3ft in front of your eyes and practice Observation of the Breath for a few minutes until you feel your respiration and heartbeat become slower and more steady. Open your eyes and gaze steadily at the flame for about two minutes. Try not to stare vacantly into space or allow your attention to wander; the idea is to remain focused as you gaze intently at the flame so that its image becomes completely absorbing. Blink as often as you need to and close your eyes if they begin to water.

Dismiss all intruding thoughts and concentrate solely on the flame. After two or three minutes, close your eyes and endeavor to retain the image of the flame in as much detail as possible; try not to let your mind wander. If the image begins to fade, open your eyes and gaze briefly at the flame again to sharpen your mental image, then resume your practice. As your concentration improves, lengthen the time for which you practice.

CLEANSING YOUR MIND AND BODY Performing *tratak* causes the eyes to water and this cleanses the tear ducts. Like *kapalabhati* (see page 83) it is considered to be one of the six traditional yogic purification practices that are collectively known as *kriyas*. Having trained your mind to a concentrated point, you are now progressing to the seventh limb of yoga: meditation.

91

Meditation

Dhayana

Meditation is sometimes described as "the space between two thoughts" because it brings a sense of mental stillness coupled with an intense awareness; the mind is at peace, yet highly alert. This distinguishes the meditative state from inactivity, where the mind simply wanders.

Only when your thoughts are calmed and focused is the mind capable of the meditative state. This allows you to benefit from feeling relaxed while also bringing a heightened sense of awareness and perception. Correct practice imparts a feeling of internal power, promotes physical and emotional rejuvenation, and can eventually lead to a state of atonement ("at-one-ness") with your entire being. This is *samadhi* or absorption, the ultimate goal of yoga.

Among the many techniques used in yoga to focus the mind are visualization (an imagined journey or narrative thought process), the use of visual stimuli such as a *yantra* or candle flame (see page 91), and the repetition of a particular phrase or sound. This phrase is called a *mantra*, and it may be a meaningful personal or devotional affirmation or simply a resonant syllable that is used to phase out distracting external noises and disturbing thoughts.

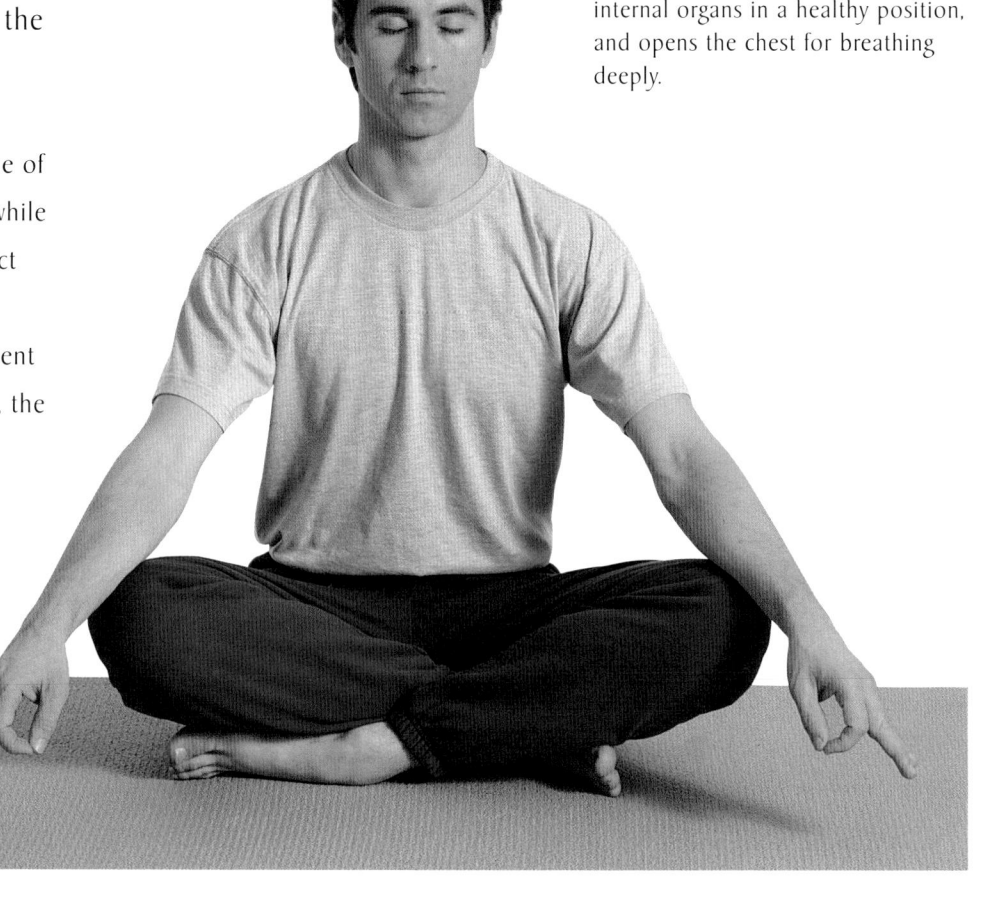

EASY POSE
This cross-legged position is easy to maintain and is ideal for meditation. It keeps the spine erect, holds the internal organs in a healthy position, and opens the chest for breathing deeply.

92

CHOOSING A MANTRA The classic Hindu or yogic *mantra* is the sacred syllable Om, used for both its significance as a reference to the absolute (or god) and the soothing, resonant quality of the sound itself. It has been practiced by students of yoga for thousands of years as an aid to meditation because it is highly effective for relieving stress and anxiety, promoting emotional well-being, heightening awareness of the body, and improving one's powers of concentration. But there are many different types of *mantra* and you by no means have to use a traditionally devotional phrase. You may feel more comfortable repeating an affirmative phrase that has a personal significance or simply a sound that you find satisfying to pronounce. Any of these *mantras* will help you attune to the correct state of mind for meditation.

HOW TO USE A MANTRA Begin by sitting comfortably in a position that you will be able to maintain without difficulty for some time and that will allow you to breathe deeply. You may lie in the Corpse Pose (see page 8) if you wish, but stay alert: this position may make you too drowsy to meditate effectively. An ideal posture for meditation is *Padmasana*, popularly known as the Lotus Position, because it is physically balanced and grounded and encourages an equivalent equilibrium in the mind. However, it does require a great deal of flexibility in the joints to maintain it properly. Even if your limbs are supple you may need to practice yoga for some time before it becomes possible, let alone comfortable, to hold after some minutes of meditation. Good alternatives are the Half Lotus Pose and *Sukhasana*, the Easy Pose (see page 10).

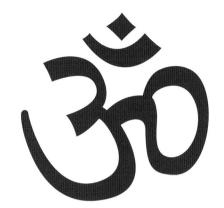

SACRED SYLLABLE
Om is the classic yoga *mantra*. It is valued for both its rich vibrational quality and its philosophical meaning, which encompasses the concept of the absolute. The Sanskrit character designating *Om* is often used as a *yantra* on which the meditator may gaze in order to anchor the mind to the abstract concept that the symbol represents.

Practice observing your breath (see pages 90–1) for a few minutes. Once your breathing is calm, divide each exhalation into two halves. To use the traditional Om *mantra*, intone the sound "oh" in a steady and quietly audible tone during the first half of each out-breath. There should be energy in the sound and it should be spoken slowly and deliberately, without becoming weak or wavering. At the half-way point of your exhalation, close your lips to produce the sound "mmm" in the same low tone. Do not allow the sound to trail off as you finish your exhalation; listen to and feel the sensations of the sound as it resonates through your body. Without pausing, inhale slowly and deeply and continue repeating the *mantra* until it is no longer a conscious effort to do so.

With practice, you may be able to concentrate on a *mantra* silently in your head, although at first it is easier to focus the mind by actually pronouncing the sound. After a few minutes, open your eyes, extend your legs, and rest for a few moments before rising.

93

Healthy Body, Healthy Mind

A balanced diet will perfectly complement your yoga practice. Yogic texts stress that the foods you consume are just as important for your health as keeping physically fit, for by following a wholesome, nutritious diet you are respecting your body and ensuring that it is in peak condition to support the activities of your mind. What's more, fueled by all the nutrients and food energy you eat, your body will stay healthy, supple, and free from disease.

94

A healthy, yogic diet and attitude to food will not only make it easier for you to perform the *asanas* in this book, it will enhance your general health *whatever* form of physical exercise you take. In yogic terms the best diet to follow is, quite simply, the most natural. This means receiving your sustenance from foods with the highest life force or *prana*. Foods that are found in a typically vegetarian diet have a high life force. The goodness gained from eating meat, fish, and poultry is considered to be far inferior in *pranic* value to that of natural foods, and is also thought to make the body stiffer.

According to yoga principles, *how* you eat is just as important as *what* you eat. So, as well as cooking with natural foods, be sure to eat slowly, regularly, and in peace—and avoid snacking between meals or overeating.

SUPPORTING YOUR YOGA PRACTICE
Your diet not only provides the physical energy to fuel your yoga workout: by supplying your body with pure foods you can concentrate more easily on your inner development, too.

THE THREE GUNAS In yoga philosophy, energy has three qualities. These are known as the *gunas* and consist of *sattvas* or purity, *rajas* or overactivity, and *tamas* or inertia. Each of us is dominated by a certain *guna*, although this may vary during different periods of our lives. Our predominant *guna* is reflected in our thoughts and behavior. For example, if you are lethargic and lacking in energy or motivation, *tamas* predominates. If you are stressed, live life at a frantic pace, and find it difficult to relax, *rajas* predominates. Practitioners of yoga seek to enhance *sattvas*, the purest form of energy, which brings mental clarity and emotional calm, and soothes and nourishes the body.

THE SATTVIC DIET This ideal regime contains the least impurities and pollutants, and therefore the highest life force or *prana*. *Sattvic* foods include fresh vegetables and fruits, beans, pulses, seeds, nuts, wholegrains, wholemeal bread, pasta, cheese, milk, butter, tofu, and honey. A *sattvic* diet is essentially a vegetarian diet. Serious yoga practitioners follow these dietary rules, but simply aiming for a healthier balance by cutting down on processed snacks, and eating regularly and not excessively can bring great improvements to your yoga practice. Improved *asanas* will help to relieve any problems connected with your digestive system, working to promote general good health.

TAMASIC FOODS TO AVOID *Tamas* is related to idleness, apathy, and ignorance. Too much *tamasic* food weakens the immune system and leads to exhaustion and negative emotions of anger and greed. Such foods include meat, onions, garlic, vinegar, alcohol, tobacco, and overripe or stale foods. Depressants such as alcohol create inertia, as does overeating (especially of foods that are high in protein such as meat, fish, or eggs). Foods that are artificially preserved, stale, burned, or grown without sunlight (such as mushrooms and root vegetables) are also considered to be *tamasic* and should therefore be kept to a minimum.

CUTTING BACK ON RAJASIC FOODS *Rajas* energy makes the mind restless, distracted, and uneasy. Because it can cause physical distress, it is an obstacle to the physical control required to practice yoga postures. Over-stimulating foods such as tea and coffee, or highly refined foods such as chocolate and other processed snacks (like potato chips) are considered *rajasic* because they produce short rushes of energy followed by a slump, therefore providing empty calories that have no nutritional value. Cut out *rajasic* foods that are excessively spicy, bitter, sour, or salty, and herbs and spices with an overpowering flavor. Certain bad habits, such as overeating, are thought to be *rajasic*, so avoid these too.

SATTVIC FOODS
These wholesome, natural foods are the most suitable for yoga practice. They are easily digested and pass through the body quickly, leaving you feeling nourished and well balanced, both physically and mentally.

INDEX

ACKNOWLEDGMENTS
Carroll & Brown would very much like to thank:
Dr Amanda Roberts for checking anatomical illustrations; Nicholas Rowe for modeling; Bettina Graham for hair and make-up; Mark Langridge for photographic assistance; Sandra Schneider for picture research.

PICTURE CREDITS
p. 6: Reed International Books Ltd; p. 87: Allan Eaton/Ancient Art and Architecture; p. 89: illustration by Jane Craddock-Watson; p. 91: illustration by Paul Williams.